# the just chill baby
# sleep book

I have collected some quotes from some of the parents I have helped in recent years. These illustrate the impact that good sleep can have on your relationships and your family.

*'Sleep training saved our lives, and our marriage. We argued constantly due to the sleep deprivation that we were experiencing. You have saved our family.'*

*'My partner and I now have the evenings to ourselves, which is just amazing. We no longer feed baby to sleep so her dad is able to put her to bed, and we can go out if we want to! The time we have together as a couple has made us feel like "us" again.'*

*'The happiness that I felt when my baby did settle (despite my doubts!) was profound. It improved our relationship.'*

*'Working on sleep ended up being the best decision that we could have made for our family. We are all happier and healthier for it.'*

*'We are going on our first date night since the baby was born, knowing that he won't wake two hours after going to bed. This has changed our lives.'*

# the just chill baby sleep book

### easy & empowering sleep solutions

## ROSEY DAVIDSON

1

Vermilion, an imprint of Ebury Publishing
20 Vauxhall Bridge Road
London SW1V 2SA

Vermilion is part of the Penguin Random House group of companies
whose addresses can be found at global.penguinrandomhouse.com

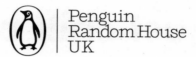

First published by Vermilion in 2023

www.penguin.co.uk

A CIP catalogue record for this book is available from the British Library

ISBN 9781785044182

The information in this book has been compiled as general guidance on infant sleeping.
It is not a substitute and not to be relied on for medical advice. So far as the author is
aware the information given is correct and up to date as at December 2022. Practice,
laws and regulations all change and the reader is encouraged to obtain up to
date professional advice on any such issues. The author and publishers disclaim,
as far as the law allows, any liability arising directly or indirectly from the use or
misuse of the information contained in this book.

Typeset in 11/15.5 pt Baskerville MT Pro by Jouve (UK), Milton Keynes
Printed and bound in Great Britain by Clays Ltd, Elcograf S.p.A.

The authorised representative in the EEA is Penguin Random House Ireland,
Morrison Chambers, 32 Nassau Street, Dublin D02 YH68

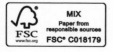

*For my babies, who made me a mum; my husband*
*(my ally in life and in parenting); my dad (the voice of reason);*
*my mum (the eternal optimist); and the friends who believed*
*in me — you know who you are. And for all those parents*
*who feel tired and alone, I've got you.*

# CONTENTS

# INTRODUCTION

This is the book that I wish I could have read when I had my first baby. When I was pregnant for the first time, I really truly believed that I was going to be an earth mother, that my baby and I would be joined together as one entity, and that we would breastfeed and sleep and be in love. Yes, we fell in love with one another, but no one can really prepare you for the sleep deprivation of those early days with a newborn (which personally hit me like a tonne of bricks!). It felt so hopeless back then – like I was inept at being a parent, all because this beautiful little squirming, squeaking being didn't seem to want to sleep.

I needed a guide like this to tell me what I am going to tell you – you don't have to deal with sleep deprivation long term. You haven't made a mistake having a baby. Your baby is not broken. Baby sleep isn't mystical. There's not one secret, no magic wand, but there is straightforward, actionable advice within the pages of this book that will set you on a path towards a more settled night's sleep.

I am so pleased you are reading this book. It is going to change how you think about baby sleep, give you practical solutions to your sleep struggles and empower you to make decisions about your little one's sleep. You might be in a fog of sleepless nights or maybe you have a bundle of joy on the way; either way, you are in the right place.

## CUTTING THROUGH THE NOISE

As soon as that blue line appears on the pregnancy test stick, there is an immense pressure to 'get it right'. There will be well-meaning comments and questions about what kind of parent you are going to be. Are you going to breastfeed or formula feed? What buggy will you get? Will you use disposable or reusable nappies? But it is baby sleep that is an obsession for so many and, once your baby is born, I can guarantee it won't be long before you are asked the ever-annoying question, 'How is your baby sleeping?'

Sleep is a controversial area – there are so many opinions and so much conflicting information out there, both in the mainstream media and online. We have never had so much information at our fingertips since the beginning of time, so why is it still so confusing? It shouldn't have to be. I am going to cut through the noise (and man, is it noisy out there), with evidence- and practice-based information and practical tips for you to get a settled night's sleep for all your family.

I believe it's less about what you 'should' do and more about what you 'could' do. You don't have to 'cry it out', but you also don't have to 'wait it out' and do nothing.

---

Nothing is set in stone, no decision is final and you can always change your mind. There is no exam at the end of parenthood, just a little person who loves you unconditionally.

---

## EMPOWERING YOU

I want to empower you with choice – to present you with options. We are all human, and I truly believe that, when it comes to humans, there is no black-and-white rule book, especially for our babies. Their needs change, our family dynamics change, life gets in the way. We need to be practical, but also flexible in our approach to parenting.

You might be surprised to hear me say that I am not your baby's expert – that only you know your baby best. No one can truly prepare you for how it feels to become a parent for the first time, but if I can teach you anything it's to trust your own gut and intuition over anything I write here, or anyone writes elsewhere.

> I want to help you to tune into your innate parental instinct and work out what your baby truly needs.

I know you are tired and you are busy, so I'm going to keep it simple. You won't find any confusing jargon or complicated sleep graphs here. Helping families to sleep is what I do, and I hope through this book I can do that for you too.

## Helping you understand

Parenting is hard, but sleep deprivation makes it even harder, and my hope is that by understanding how we sleep and the importance of sleep to our health and well-being, you may be a little bit kinder to yourself. Sleep truly is the elixir of life – it affects every fibre of our being – so when our little humans come into this world it can be a bit of a shock (to say the least!) when our sleep is disrupted. But you do not need to be sleep-deprived long term. It might feel hard right now because it *is* hard.

I am going to explain how sleep works in a simple way so that you can understand what this lovely shut-eye is all about. Note that I am not a neuroscientist, nor a scientist, but the things I will talk about are grounded in science. The science is the science, but my expertise comes in the 'doing' part – the actionable advice to help you get more sleep.

## Providing answers and guidance

'Why does getting my baby to sleep sometimes feel like an impossible mountain to climb?' 'Why, when I thought I had it nailed, has my baby suddenly stopped sleeping?' 'Why have my baby's two-hour naps turned into micro naps?' 'Does my baby even need a two-hour nap?' I am asked all these questions and many more like them on a daily basis. Sleep can feel incredibly hard for many reasons, but the answers to how we approach it don't have to be. I know you want practical answers, so that's what I am going to give you. I am not a magician (despite being referred to as such on more than one occasion), but I know baby sleep. I know how hard it is when you are sleep-deprived (I have been there myself) and I also know how hard it is to find the answers you are looking for.

Many people ask me whether they have ruined their baby by rocking/feeding/sshing [insert other settling method here!] to sleep and if it is too late to change this. The answer is no! If your baby's sleep has been broken up until now, don't worry – your baby won't be damaged, and you are certainly in good company. I wouldn't have built the business that I have if it wasn't for parents needing help with sleep and if I wasn't able to help them. The countless families whose lives have been transformed by my simple, actionable advice are the proof of the pudding. From here on in you can work on prioritising sleep, and the health of you and your family.

From birth to our oldest age, there are things we can do to optimise our sleep. Babyhood is where it all starts and where I am going to help you set off on the right track. As your little one grows, the opportunity to improve sleep and practise the methods in this book will present itself. These methods are about finding what works for your baby – their preferences and sensitivities – and giving them the very best opportunity to fall asleep and get the best night that they can.

## OUR LITTLE HUMANS

Babies are not robots – they are their own little biological beings whose needs ebb and flow like a tide as they grow. It can be hard to make sense of what is going on and to keep up with their rapid growth and changes in this first year. Having said that, they do have a lot in common with one another. They might not reach them at the same time, but they have similar milestones and stages, and similar needs. So, while each baby is different, they all feel very familiar to me. There are patterns and needs that I have noticed in my years of practice, continued learning and, of course, from being a mum to my three little wonders.

Each of the babies and children I have helped has been different in many ways, but the simple principles I apply to each sleep challenge are the same. While each parent and baby dynamic has taught me something new, I always find similarities in their sleep challenges.

Finding what works for you and your baby is the challenge, and that is why we are here.

## SUPPORTING YOU

I am here to support you and hopefully be a guiding light in your first year of parenthood. I want you to feel calm and confident about your baby's sleep. To try to be the best parent you can be is admirable, but know that your best is always good enough. Don't let anyone else tell you otherwise. You know your limits; you know how you deal with things. You are doing the best you can with what you have.

I am going to explain how sleep works in a simple way so that you can understand what this lovely shut-eye is all about. Note that I am not a doctor, nor a neuroscientist, nor a scientist, but the things I will talk about are grounded in science. The science is the science, but my expertise comes in the *doing* part, the actionable advice – based on my lived experiences and consultancy work – to help you get more sleep.

If your situation is unsustainable and you have reached out for this book, then you have taken the first step in admitting you need a little help, and you can be proud of that. The hardest part is admitting to yourself that things are unmanageable – to let go of the overwhelming feeling that you should be able to do it all yourself, that you should be able to cope, that you are failing. You are not failing; the system has failed you. You haven't been taught about these things. Your baby didn't come with an instruction manual. We are all human and we are all designed to have a support network in place. For those of you who don't have that or who need a voice to advocate for you, I hope this book is going to be that for you.

## ME AND MY JOURNEY

I am a mother of three beautiful children, who all sleep really well. I run a sleep consultancy, with a team of outstanding women behind me. But it wasn't always like this. My first baby was a challenge. It was the first time I had ever experienced real sleep deprivation and, as I said, it hit me like a tonne of bricks. That, combined with struggling to breastfeed, recovering from birth and generally getting to grips with my new identity as a mother, was a challenge. I do think that, for all of us, there is this period of intense change and adaptation, and, although some will seemingly sail through this period, most of us find it tricky.

My daughter wasn't a terrible sleeper and, in fact, for the first couple of months (after we sorted out her feeding issues), I was coping. But then it all changed, and I wasn't coping anymore. The wakes became more and more frequent, she became more and more fractious, and I was left a shell of my former self. I couldn't operate anymore. I didn't want to see anyone or talk to anyone, and I cried a lot. I convinced myself that there must have been something wrong with her, that she must have developed some underlying illness for sleep to be this bad. It turns out that everything was just upside down, inside out and totally and utterly solvable.

I had read all the baby books when I was pregnant for the first time, but none of them seemed to help me. They all felt so complicated and contradictory, with strange rules and stipulations that didn't have any logic or evidence to back them up.

I needed to talk to someone, urgently. I went to see my GP and health visitor, and I also spoke to an 'old-school' nanny. What all of them seemed to hone in on was routine and how she settled herself. I took steps to work on sleep myself – I looked at her routine with the help of my health visitor and the nanny, and realised I was trying to force her to nap when she wasn't ready and that I wasn't giving her the space she needed to settle herself off to sleep. I was suffocating her. Every whimper, moan or movement, I was on high alert, jumping up and out of bed to soothe her.

She hit six months and it was time, time for change. We worked out a really good rhythm to our days – I was no longer trying to force her to sleep when she wasn't tired. She was a totally different baby – an absolute joy! And I bloomed into the mother I had always wanted to be. By giving her the space that she needed, she learned how to get herself to sleep, and stay asleep throughout the night. Of course, we have had bumps in the road with illness, but this little girl loves sleep. She taught me how to do what I do and she is the reason that I am writing this book right now. Our journey inspired me to help others and gave me a thirst for knowledge about sleep. I did my research, got a qualification and the rest is history.

Two more babies have since come along and, while they are different and totally individual, I applied what I had learned over the years and they both slept soundly from a much younger age.

Funnily enough, I wrote this book across the course of the first year of my youngest child's life. I followed every twist and turn of his early months as the pages of this book were born.

---

I want to give this gift to you, the gift of a good night's sleep. Good sleep shouldn't be a secret. It shouldn't be complicated.

---

Thank you for reaching out and grabbing this book. I hope it can be a lifeline for you, one I could have done with way back when.

## MY APPROACH

As you work through this book, you will see that I don't believe in a one-size-fits-all approach. Every baby, parent and family is different, so it's important that we adapt our methods and our expectations accordingly. This isn't about absolutes or magic routines that are the same for each baby.

---

There are similarities between our babies and things that commonly work, but part of the journey is working out which parts suit you and which don't.

---

The power comes in knowing the basics of how we can change things if our situation becomes unsustainable, and how to navigate those early weeks, months and the first year. My suggestions are based on evidence, but also my own clinical practice and what I have noticed over the years. One of the things that I always tell parents is that anything goes, *as long as it is working for you*. I want you to feel empowered, confident and equipped to tune into your parental instinct.

# HOW TO USE THIS BOOK

The chapters are designed to be read in the order in which they appear, but you can also dip in and out and refer back to the sections you need at the time.

**Part 1:** Discover why sleep is essential to your health and well-being, as well as your baby's, and become empowered to give your baby the best start in life through good sleep.

**Part 2:** Get the basics right: from where your baby will sleep, to which bedding to use and the all-important safe sleeping guidance. Discover what to expect in the early days and months to help you maximise your own and your baby's sleep and begin putting an early routine in place if you want to.

**Part 3:** Prepare yourself for the four-to-six-month progression as your baby's sleep patterns change. Discover the sleep-training methods that will help you make informed choices about how to help your baby sleep.

**Part 4:** Equip yourself to deal with any of the challenges that might disrupt your baby's sleep, such as travelling, a change of childcare and your baby being ill. Prepare for how the transition back to work may affect your baby's sleep and how sleep difficulties may impact your relationships.

Finally, at the back of the book, dip into the common Q&As that have enabled me to help countless clients with their sleep concerns.

It is important to me that you can keep using this as a guide throughout the first year of your baby's life, and especially that you turn to it when you need a helping hand. I have chosen the topics that are close to my heart, but also those that I have seen time and time again in my practice. Each family dynamic is different, and you will see different challenges from those of your friends' and family's babies.

The book is designed to cover the basics of sleep, while also helping you to adapt the information to your unique situation. You will find some similar themes running through the book that are the keystones to a good night's sleep.

Think of this book like a bag of tricks you will carry with you across this first year. We have the foundations, which are the sturdy material it is made of, the straps to carry you when things get tough, and the tools and tips inside for you to dip in and out of along your journey.

I can't wait to metaphorically hold your hand on this journey. So, let's get down to business and work on making life a bit more manageable.

# PART 1

# 1

# GOOD SLEEP IS NON-NEGOTIABLE!

Let me start by saying that wanting to establish better sleep for your baby so that you can get more sleep yourself is *not* selfish (I've lost count of the number of times parents have started an enquiry with 'I know it's selfish, but . . .'). Your sleep matters!

---

Looking after your sleep is looking after yourself so you can look after your baby, your family and maintain the relationships in your life, not to mention your career, your social life and other interests.

---

Parenting is hard. We can feel overwhelmed, stressed and pulled in every direction. Throw in sleep deprivation and you've got a recipe for burnout.

You may be familiar with the analogy of putting on your own oxygen mask first. You will, in fact, have heard this if you have ever flown in an aeroplane. I remember the first time we flew with my eldest and I couldn't imagine ever being able to do that – the thought of her sitting there helpless while I put my oxygen mask on. But then I thought to myself, *What on earth are you thinking? It makes total sense. What use would I be to her if I passed out because I couldn't breathe, and she was left alone?*

It is no different in our day-to-day lives. We may not be in mortal danger and need an oxygen mask, but the collated toll of hours, days, weeks and months of sleep deprivation will get to you – the days when your eyes sting, when you feel like you've made a mistake, when you crash your car. These are just things I have been told by families who I have helped over the years. There are so many more stories out there.

My point is this: how can you look after your baby and be at your very best when you are sleep-deprived? It is not selfish to want the basic human requirement of some sleep. Of course, *some* sleep disturbance is normal in small children. None of us strictly sleep solidly through the night. It's normal for babies to wake regularly and feed (especially in the early days) and it can feel relentless, but there comes a point when we can start practising the art of falling asleep without so much parental intervention. There does come a point when more restorative sleep is possible.

## OUR SLEEP NEEDS

Let's not forget that every adult has a slightly different tolerance for sleep deprivation.

Some of us need more sleep than others. I am a 'high sleep needs' adult, for example. To function at my very best, that means getting eight to nine hours (I think this is why I got into the business – my thirst for sleep gave me a thirst for information on the topic!). My husband only needs seven hours to be bright as a button.

Whatever our individual sleep needs, we need to be hitting a decent amount of rest to be mentally and physically capable of looking after other people. If we neglect that, I truly believe we leave ourselves open to illness, both physical and mental. Mental illness is more complex than this of course – many types of mental illness cause sleep deprivation themselves, but many are exacerbated by lack of sleep. It is a bit of a chicken-and-egg situation – one where prioritising your rest always wins.

## TIME FOR YOU

Making time for yourself is important. We can sometimes feel totally lost when we become parents and we spend every bit of free time trying to catch up on sleep. I am a huge fan of daytime napping (done in the right way; I'll get on to this!), but you don't want to spend every waking hour trying to catch up on lost sleep when you could be relaxing, reading a book, working out or just sitting and enjoying some silence. It is not selfish to want to enjoy a meal in peace with your partner. It is not selfish to want to have a bath on your own, with the sound of the water lapping on your skin as your only company.

I'm not saying this is easy. It took me about four weeks after my third baby to have the time to take a bath – the time without him feeding and without my other children needing me. I distinctly remember the feeling – the first time I think I truly relaxed in four weeks, while he slept supervised by my husband. Even that 20-minute bath felt like a holiday. Everything is relative, right? If you've had a baby on you 24/7 for four weeks and you get a break like that, it can be enough to rejuvenate you.

## YOUR SLEEP ROUTINE

Sometimes changing our baby's sleep habits means that we need to address our own. Looking inwards at our own 'sleep hygiene', and attitudes and beliefs around sleep, is often key to this. Many of us are resistant to having a regular routine, but the science does not lie. We are not designed to stay up late at night when it's dark – we have modern technology to thank for that habit. We are supposed to get up early and get on with our days. We are naturally routine-led mammals. Modern life has in many ways made us forget how to work with our biology. We are supposed to get lots of exposure to natural light. We are more relaxed, productive and at ease when we have a predictable rhythm to our days.

We are juggling so much nowadays. Social media and being reachable 24/7 means we are constantly switched on, constantly comparing. We are trying to raise our babies, hold down a job, have a clean home, make healthy food, keep fit *and* have a baby who sleeps well. It is no wonder that parents are burnt out, over-whelmed and confused.

---

Getting back to basics with our babies and prioritising rest can be totally transformative. Those everyday tasks that feel impossible when you are tired suddenly become a bit easier to manage.

---

## YOUR RELATIONSHIP WITH SLEEP

This is perhaps the most important thing to think about. How do you view your sleep? Is it something you push to the bottom of your list of priorities? Do you feel like you are too busy to get to bed early? Do you feel like it is selfish to want to protect your sleep or to get more of it? These preconceived ideas that we have about what it is to be a good parent are dangerous – that we should sac-rifice years of good sleep for our children, when in fact a tired parent isn't helpful to them either (they need a well-slept, positive and healthy parent). Of course, there are times we are going to be tired, and we need to expect a level of sleep disruption when we have a baby, but it shouldn't be long term.

Taking the time to work on our own sleep almost feels

decadent in our society, when it really shouldn't be – it's far more fashionable to talk about a new healthy-eating regime or joining a gym. So why do we feel so icky about it? Often when we become parents our own sleep needs become an afterthought. We spend so much time focusing on our babies that we don't prioritise our rest.

Saying that you want more sleep or are working on your own sleep doesn't translate as 'I'm not a good parent'; it just means you are working on a huge influencer on your health and happiness. Sleep helps us in all aspects of our lives, but especially our relationships. Sleep deprivation can make us feel lonely and less likely to reach out and forge new friendships, and to look after the ones we have. When we sleep well, we can feel more empathy for our partners, friends and family, and can find the everyday interactions with people we meet to be more positive.

---

Treating yourself with the care with which you treat your baby is a starting point – by making sure you are well fed, happy and rested. Sleep is not a luxury.
It's a necessity.

---

## YOUR ATTITUDE TO SLEEP

There are a few things that I want you to think about when it comes to your own set of rules. The truth is we never know exactly how we are going to feel about things until we are in the thick of it. Some of you may be reading this book before your baby has arrived, and some of you may be reading this while your baby is napping, or some of you might be desperately trying to help yourself out of a sleep crisis.

Whatever your position is now, it can help you to think about and reflect on the questions below. It is an interesting exercise to refer back to your answers once you have finished this book and again once you have worked on your baby's sleep. See if your outlook and belief system have shifted at all.

- What was your own sleep like as a child? Do you have any memories of your bedtime routine?
- What are your own sleep needs like? Do you need a lot of sleep to feel well?
- What is your relationship like with sleep now? Is your bed a sanctuary? Do you have a good bedtime routine or do you just crash?
- Do you like routine or do you prefer to take things as they come?
- Are you prepared to change how you do things to prioritise your baby?
- Do you have a good support network to help you rest/clean/eat?
- What kind of temperament does your baby have? Are they easy-going? Are they sensitive?
- What would you like to achieve by working on your little one's sleep (better naps, a full night's sleep or fewer wakings, for example)?
- What would be your ideal outcome from working through this book?
- What are your hopes for your little one's sleep in the future?
- Do you and your partner have different attitudes to both your own sleep and what you want for your baby? (See Chapter 11 for more on relationships and sleep.)

## MODERN-DAY PRESSURES

Modern life has a lot to answer for. Things have changed – we don't have the 'villages' of old, the network of family members, grandparents, cousins and aunties and uncles all on our doorstep. Many parents are socially isolated. It may be that one parent is home alone taking care of the baby with no family nearby. This can make caring for your baby and dealing with lack of sleep even harder. Modern lifestyles mean we are constantly multitasking. We have more to do than ever before and we are juggling it all with looking after a small person.

There are other things at play too – the dangerous narrative that we should become martyrs for our children; that they should never feel sadness, never whimper, moan or groan, or experience time in their own company. We will never be able to provide the perfect home, be the perfect parent or produce the perfect child, because perfect doesn't exist.

---

Being a good-enough parent is good enough. Your baby can grow up to be a well-balanced individual, without needing to be physically attached to you 24/7.

---

## SHARING THE CARE

I have written this book to be inclusive of all parents and families, whatever they look like. Although things are changing for many families (I have met families where the care – and the sleep deprivation! – is entirely shared), for most it still comes down to one parent, perhaps because that parent happens to be breastfeeding the baby or because the other parent is the main breadwinner. Either way, it seems a little unfair.

It only seems to be recently that there has been a shift in our social consciousness, a recognition that parenting is a full-time job. It is not mucking around at home enjoying parental leave, doing yoga and baking. It can be the most challenging period of our lives. To sustain a small person who has constant needs that only we can attend to is exhausting. It's beautiful but exhausting (and you are allowed to say that too, without feeling guilty).

I truly believe that, if it is possible in the dynamic of your family, it's hugely beneficial to share the load a little. Even if that means you get one lie-in a week, one night off or your partner gets up with baby in the mornings – whatever it takes so that you can feel there is some sort of shared care. If you don't have a partner, then I urge you to enlist the help of a friend or family member to give you a break. You don't need to feel guilty about asking for or accepting this help either. You don't need to spend that time cleaning or cooking. You do what you damn well want to – if that's watching Netflix while eating ice cream in your pyjamas, so be it. Hell, if it's doing some yoga, going for a walk or flicking through magazines at the supermarket, that's okay too.

### Redressing the balance

*I remember a couple I worked with a few years ago. The dad worked long hours in the city in a demanding job and the mum had worked in a fast-paced advertising agency before going on maternity leave. I went to visit the mum at home when their baby, David, had just turned six months. When she opened the door to me, she broke down and fell into my arms crying. She then apologised profusely. She told me how lonely she was, and there was an overwhelming sense of relief that she could share how she was feeling with someone. They didn't have any family close by and none of their friends had babies. She had gone from being in a client-facing role, in which she dressed in designer gear head to toe and wore flawless make-up, to seeing me in her dressing gown with no* make-up on and her hair unwashed for a week. I reassured her that she was not the only one to cry on my shoulder, and absolutely not the first parent I had seen in their dressing gown.

I got to know both David and his mum during my visit, and we worked on a strategy to improve his sleep and his routine, but the main thing we spoke about was how the balance was off in their home. Her husband got up and went to work and wasn't involved with the burden of sleep deprivation. She did all the night-time settling and spent all day with David on her own. She had become very quiet and introverted, when she was an extrovert and a naturally sociable person at heart.

We looked at her partner's timings and decided that, on the days when he could, he would get up with David and have him for a minimum of 30 minutes while she had an extra bit of sleep, or a shower, or a cup of tea, or whatever. This still gave the dad time to make his train, but she got a moment of quiet to be herself. Thirty minutes doesn't sound long, but even knowing she had that window of time helped her feel better and prepared for her day.

At the weekend, they would take it in turns to have a lie-in. Her partner agreed to settle David one night a week if he woke during the night, and to let her sleep. Although he was at work during my visit, we video-called him on his lunch break and worked this out. They had a chat that evening and she explained exactly how she had been feeling. The overwhelming sense of responsibility for David's sleep felt like a weight she couldn't bear on her own. She felt like she had lost part of her identity as a professional person too. We spoke about how, as soon as she felt up to it, she would have a morning, afternoon or evening out to herself – whether this was a coffee at a local coffee shop, an afternoon at a spa or an evening with a friend. It turns out that two weeks later David was sleeping through the night and Mum was ready to go out for the day and evening with her old work colleagues. She felt rested *and supported to do so. Although David's sleep was key in this process, feeling supported by her partner and helping to share the load allowed her that bit of head space to regain her confidence and some of her sense of self again.*

## COMMUNICATING YOUR NEEDS

It can be tricky if one parent is getting more sleep than the other. Perhaps you are breastfeeding and taking on all nights, or perhaps your partner works and you've decided between you that you will take the lion's share. Looking after your baby is also a job – a full-time one. You both need sleep to do your jobs, so coming to an agreement about the division of domestic chores, and sleep, can make things smoother. There is, however, such a thing as competitive tiredness. So many couples argue about who got a worse night's sleep, whose turn it is to get up with the baby and who feels worse the next day. It is hard not to get drawn into a negative spiral here. Saying 'I am tired' does not mean that the other person is not tired. It's okay for you and your partner to say you are tired. It's okay to report to your partner how many times you were woken in the night, but it's better to use that energy to make a positive plan. Even if your partner is working and you are at home, you still need to sleep. Perhaps you have decided that their sleep needs to be prioritised for them to work (which is entirely valid if that is how your family dynamic works), but even just knowing that on one or two mornings a week you get to catch up and have a lie-in can make a world of difference.

- Have an honest but calm conversation, explaining that you are both doing a job and that some support and recognition would make you feel valued and cared for.
- How could you approach things differently to support your family's sleep?
- Can you create a rota where you take it in turns to get up with baby?

---

It's okay to report to your partner how many times you were woken in the night, but it's better to use that energy to make a positive plan.

## DOING WHAT'S RIGHT FOR YOU AND YOUR FAMILY

Some people choose to 'ride out' sleep challenges, but not everyone has that privilege. All families look different and have a different set of priorities, beliefs and cultures. Some are better set up to focus solely on the care of their babies with no other responsibilities. Some of those families may find it easier to wait it out. Some of you reading this might be in the same situation as those families and still want to improve sleep – that is also okay. You don't need to feel guilty about your feelings about your little one's sleep. Each family I have worked with over the years has been different, but they all have something in common – they are reaching out for help, just as you have reached out to read this book. Do not let others dictate how you experience struggle. It's okay to find it hard and to want to change it. Keep in mind that what one family might see as a problem, another wouldn't – perhaps they have slightly different tolerance levels or different expectations. Everyone has a different threshold for what they can handle in terms of sleep disruption.

There is nothing wrong with having a baby who goes to bed before you, not only so that you get some time for yourself but so they get the sleep that they require within a 24-hour period. Kids need more sleep than us, and babies need even more. To get it all in, I believe that they need an earlier bedtime than us.

Another, equally important reason for wanting your baby to go to bed in the evening is for their own well-being. I truly believe that most babies – even as newborns (with the exception being the early weeks when they have things a bit upside down) – and children will be happier if they are in bed by 8pm, and I also believe that, as parents, we end up happier as a result. Yes, they will wake regularly for feeding when they are little, but a lot of evening fussiness can be put down to them telling you they want to go to bed. This doesn't mean abandoning them in a room on their own. It just means putting into place a simple bedtime routine and settling them down for the night (with you), at an earlier hour. Of course, there are always exceptions to the rule – those little outliers who are happy going to bed later. And if that works for your family, it's okay too.

## Going it alone

*I once had a client who was a single mum of three children, the youngest being six months. She had no choice but to work on her baby's sleep because she ran her own business in the evenings. Her husband had left her when the baby was six weeks old – she was a stay-at-home mum, so didn't get any maternity pay. She had previously worked in the fashion industry and had always dreamed of having her own clothing line. Fast forward six months and the handmade clothes she had designed and sold on Instagram had really taken off. She was flooded with orders. Her baby wasn't sleeping, however, and she had no childcare other than her mum, who would cover one afternoon a week (she worked too).*

*When she contacted me, I was absolutely floored that she was working and getting up at 5am with her six-month-old and running her home and her older kids' lives too. She told me she had saved up for our phone call, and how important it was that we improved things. She said she started bed-sharing (when she really didn't want to be doing this!) for ease during the nights. She was so tired by the time she got to bed in the evenings (she went to bed with the baby) that she didn't have the energy to do anything else, but her baby was waking up four to five times a night and starting the day so early, she was literally broken.*

*After we worked together, she was able to put the baby down at 7.30pm, and her older kids were down by 8pm. She would feed the baby at 11pm before she went to bed, and otherwise the baby slept through in her own cot. This mum didn't have the space for baby's own room, so the cot was in her room, but we still managed it.*

*Almost overnight her productivity increased and, to this day, she has a very successful business. She was able to work flexibly around her baby, in the evenings and at naptimes. The business flourished and she was then able to afford some extra childcare with a local childminder.*

So now that we're clear that wanting your baby to sleep so that you can get more sleep, function and be a better parent is more than okay, let's understand just why sleep is so essential to our health and well-being.

# 2

# THE TRANSFORMATIVE POWER OF SLEEP

The very fact that you are reading this book probably means that you are already sold on the idea of a good night's sleep. However, I really think that the power and importance of sleep is underestimated in modern life. Sleep deprivation seems to go hand in hand with parenthood, but what does that mean for the parents? Does that mean that we sacrifice ten good years of sleep? Or even longer depending on how many children we have? The effects of this could be catastrophic to our health.

I see families every day who are totally transformed by a good night's sleep – their relationships are saved; they get back to work; and their lives become manageable again. Some tired parents seem to wear sleep deprivation as a badge of honour, making light of it, and in doing so they inadvertently project their own complicated relationship with sleep on to others. Sleep deprivation is no joke. It ruins lives, causes accidents and leaves us miserable. Yes, we may never sleep again with the reckless abandon of our pre-baby days (cue still being awake waiting for our teenagers to get home), but we can absolutely be well-rested.

You don't need to sacrifice your health and your well-being for your baby. Your baby doesn't want this

either – they also need sleep not only to survive,
but to flourish.

## SLEEP IS ESSENTIAL TO GOOD HEALTH

We need to wake up to the idea that sleep is just as important as, if not more important than, a healthy diet and daily movement. Without sleep we can't function at our best. Sleep affects every single function of our bodies. There is so much about sleep that we still don't know, but what we do know is that it is a tonic for the body. How are we supposed to look after our babies, drive a car, hold down a job and feed ourselves when we are all severely sleep-deprived? Lack of sleep leaves us vulnerable – vulnerable to illness, obesity, depression and more. It literally reduces our life expectancy. You might take a daily vitamin (if you don't then you definitely need vitamin D – see page 96), but it is restorative sleep that is the best health supplement. We need to be thinking about our daily, or rather nightly, intake of sleep just as we look at the food we are eating and the movement in our days. Professional athletes are literally prescribed naps to help their performance. Think about that for a moment.

Working on our sleep shouldn't be a luxury. We should
all be thinking about it and protecting it as we grow up
and when we grow old.

## TYPES OF SLEEP

The two basic types of sleep are REM (rapid eye movement) and non-REM, and both are equally important. How you feel when you are awake and how well your body functions daily depend on whether you are getting enough of both types.

### REM sleep

During this type of sleep your eyes move around quickly in different directions, but they are not actually sending any visual information to your brain as they do this. REM sleep is the type of sleep when you dream. The muscles of our arms and legs are paralysed during REM sleep to protect us from trying to act out our dreams. During REM sleep we link together memories and learning, a bit like laying down the small pieces of a giant intricate jigsaw puzzle. It is often why people wake up having solved a problem in their sleep! Your brain literally does the work while you rest. It is also when you are most likely to have vivid dreams – those ones where you wake up and wonder for a moment if they were real.

### Non-REM sleep

During this type of sleep our eyes don't move around. While we experience stages of light non-REM sleep during our sleep cycles – and these are where many new parents will spend a lot of their sleeping time – the most restorative non-REM sleep takes place in the deep stages, when our body is in recovery mode, when we build muscles and tissue and strengthen our immune systems. I like to think of it like restoring our 'hard drives'. This is when the brain restores and repairs the body.

It can feel hard to wake up from deep non-REM sleep – you can feel quite nauseous, groggy and disorientated if you are woken during this stage. I have been woken by my kids in non-REM sleep before and I always know because I feel goddamn awful.

Both adults and babies cycle in and out of REM and non-REM sleep, with partial wakings in between. If our conditions of sleep are consistent, we are more likely to continue sleeping than to fully rouse, but babies often wake between sleep cycles and need our assistance to fall back to sleep. On page 110 you will discover how you can work on your baby doing this!

## BODY CLOCK

We also need to be sleeping at a time that is in sync with our internal body clock (also called our circadian rhythm). In the early evening we start to produce a hormone called melatonin – sometimes called the 'vampire hormone', as it comes out after dark! It helps us to feel sleepy, and the production of this can aid sleep at bedtime. This is why you may have heard that turning off devices and artificial light in the evenings can help you get to sleep. If we don't get enough sleep, or sleep at the wrong times, we can end up feeling terrible – emotional, groggy, short-tempered and downright unwell. Our babies also need to have daily schedules in line with their internal body clock (see page 225), otherwise it's possible they could be sleepy, but still struggle to go off to sleep.

## SLEEP PRESSURE

Our 'homeostatic sleep drive' or, more simply, 'sleep pressure' is when there is an increase of the hormone adenosine in the body. Think of it like a kettle that is gradually heating up during the day and reaches boiling point at bedtime. It is our drive to sleep – that super sleepy feeling you get when you are so tired that your eyelids are dropping. The pressure builds more and more for every hour we are awake and helps us to get to sleep and stay asleep.

If you need to nap, it's best to keep it to early afternoon and for no longer than 30 minutes, otherwise it can wreak havoc on your own sleep. But – and it's a big but – if you are not getting much sleep at night due to your baby waking and are using naps to catch up in the day, then this rule is out of the window. Just grab sleep whenever you can!

When babies nap during the day it reduces sleep pressure. It is important that they do this so that they can get through to bedtime – they need regular rest during the day. However, we need to keep on top of their ever-changing 'sleep requirements' as they grow. If they nap for too long or too late then sleep pressure is not at its optimum when they go to bed at night-time.

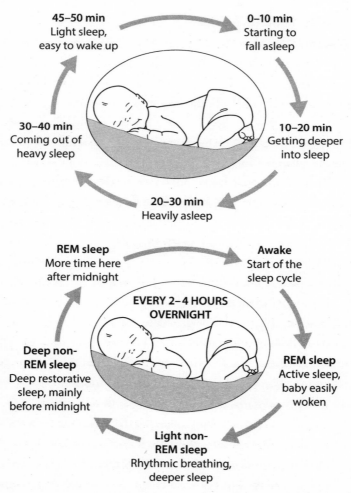

*This diagram gives you an idea of what your baby's sleep looks like, showing how they move between sleep cycles.*

Sleep pressure decreases again while we are asleep and reaches a low after a settled night's sleep. Our sleep drive can also be affected if we have had a particularly energetic day or if we are unwell and our immune system is working hard to fight something off – our sleep drive naturally adjusts to signal to us to rest up.

## FACTORS THAT AFFECT SLEEP

When you go to bed, it is important to give yourself the best chance of a good night's sleep, so check your overall sleep hygiene and make improvements where you can.

- **Artificial light:** Avoiding artificial light at least 60 minutes before bedtime is advisable. In fact, make it longer than this if you are struggling to switch off at night. The light from devices and the TV is particularly tricky for sleep – the blue light they emit tells our brains to stay awake. You can also dim the lights in your home – perhaps switch to a lamp in the evenings, or if you want to go the extra mile you could have a candlelit bath.
- **Diet:** Assess your diet. Consuming lots of processed, sugary food, alcohol and caffeine could be affecting your sleep.
- **Temperature and bedding:** Make sure your room isn't too hot as a cooler temperature is conducive to better sleep. It is preferable to sleep in a cooler room with thicker bedding, than a warmer room with light bedding. Cotton, breathable bedding is best. If you can, open a window either before you go to bed or during the night if you are awake.

- **Medication:** Some medical conditions and certain medications may be affecting your sleep. Speak to your doctor if you think this is the case.
- **Natural light:** Make sure you are getting enough exposure to natural light during the day – humans were not designed to be inside all day long. This is key to good sleep and is a simple actionable thing to build into your day. Getting out in natural light in the mornings is especially effective.

## BEWARE THE GREMLINS!

We often struggle to make healthy food choices when we are tired – our hunger hormones leptin and ghrelin are responsible for this. That's why we reach for stodgy or sugary foods when we are tired. Ghrelin levels will increase (I call it ghrelin the gremlin!) and leptin levels decrease. Leptin is the hormone responsible for keeping you full and ghrelin tells you to eat more high-calorie foods. So, if you are trying to make healthy choices, lack of sleep really won't be helping you.

Tired adults often rely on sugar and caffeine to get through the day, which in turn can impact sleep even more. I am not telling you that you can't have your much-loved cup of coffee to get you through the day, but consuming caffeine in the afternoons will impact your sleep quality well into the night. If you struggle to get back to sleep after waking with your baby, it is well worth assessing your caffeine intake across the day.

Interestingly, you will also see children become much fussier with their food when they are tired. Babies who aren't well-slept can often struggle with the process of starting solids too. They are simply too tired and grumpy to sit in a highchair and explore something new.

## A MATTER OF LIFE OR DEATH . . .

I don't want to frighten you, but the cold hard facts are that you are more likely to crash your car when you haven't slept well because your reaction times are slower. This is an extreme example, but accidents due to tiredness happen every day. It is why lorry drivers have scheduled sleep breaks – it is simply not safe enough for them to be at the wheel when they have been driving for a number of hours without sleep.

But where do parents get their scheduled breaks? We have to carve out these moments in our days ourselves; no one else can do it for us.

I just want you to know how important it is for you to prioritise your rest. I know it's not easy when we are up against so much. Modern life – screens, Netflix, and multitasking careers and family life all play a part. We are no longer simply surviving – making sure we eat, having to move to stay alive and sleep when it gets dark as our predecessors would have many years ago. We have school runs, we have jobs to get to, we have technology sending us reminders (which cleverly keep us on our phones) keeping us up at night. There is a lot more at play in today's world than being kept awake at night by our babies, even if it feels like that's the one thing keeping you awake. In an ideal world, we wouldn't have to juggle all these things – we would live in a village where we were surrounded by helpful relatives and we would have someone feeding us while we fed our babies. But this isn't real life for (most) parents nowadays.

By using this book, you will learn to recognise when you need help, how to create a support system and find ways to cope when you are the midst of a sleep crisis. I believe that, while it is never too late to work on sleep, early intervention is key when a family is really struggling.

## WHY BABIES NEED RESTFUL SLEEP

Let's not forget our babies in this equation – they need restful sleep too. We're not just trying to get our babies to sleep to benefit us. Sleeping well is essential to their growth and development.

---

When babies sleep, their brains are incredibly busy. They are processing a huge amount of information, making sense of what they have seen and learned throughout their days.

---

During the first year of their lives, they go through rapid development. Their cells are dividing and repairing tissues, and their bodies release hormones that are vital for their development. Their immune systems rely on sleep to produce white blood cells, which are especially important for when they first encounter the nasty germs of baby and toddlerhood. At each nap and bedtime, they are literally recharging their battery.

There is a huge amount of growth happening when our babies sleep – considering that they tend to triple their birth weight by 12 months old. This is why your baby may seem particularly sleepy when they are going through a growth spurt – their naps might be longer than usual and they may do longer stints at night. I am not saying that a baby who has fragmented sleep isn't going to grow and develop, because they will. It might just mean that they are not functioning at their very best. There is some research to suggest that babies who sleep well at night have an 'easier' temperament and are more adaptable, which is certainly something to consider.[1] It stands to reason that sleeping well means we are more sociable.

Some sleep disturbance is inevitable as your baby comes into this world. It is normal for them to wake often to fill their teeny tummies and to want to be close to you while they make sense of this strange new world they have been born into.

But sleeping well in babyhood and childhood will set your little one up with great sleep habits for life. I truly believe that better sleep will transform your life as a parent. Having a great predictable routine with your little one gives you the freedom to enjoy their awake times and to have a restful evening when they are asleep. We should all be able to look forward to going to bed, not dread it every night (as so many do who are suffering from disturbed sleep).

Now that we've looked at why sleep is so important, let's empower you to give your baby the best start in life through sleep.

# 3

# BECOMING EMPOWERED

I believe the key to empowering yourself as a parent is to tune into your intuition and your baby. What can get in the way of this is the tonnes of conflicting information out there, as well as the temptation to compare your situation to others (so many people will be quick to tell you what worked for them and what, in their opinion, you are doing 'wrong').

If you search online around the topic of baby sleep you will be inundated with differing opinions, methods, books and articles. If you look closely enough, you may find common themes, but so much of it is conflicting. For new parents this is mind-boggling, and some of the less reputable advice can even set you up to fail before you have even started. Much like your doctor would tell you to stop googling your health concerns, I am going to tell you to stop googling your little one's sleep. Instead, focus in on your baby, their needs and your priorities. Tune into your intuition and find what works for you. It feels like we have lost our way a little bit with all the 'rules' out there.

You don't need to do anything super extreme, but you can make solid changes to move forward and get a settled night's sleep. So many parents remain paralysed with fear over hushed conversations about the damage of sleep training, how you should never wake a sleeping baby and how they will just sleep when they are ready. Of course, you can always choose to wait it out – maybe that is sustainable for you. But if you are in an unsustainable situation, know that you can absolutely take action and do what's right for you and your family. There is always a middle ground for everything. In Chapter 8 you will find a range of methods to try out.

## MAKING THE RIGHT DECISIONS FOR YOU

One of the biggest shocks I had when I became a parent was that I realised I would have to make decisions on behalf of someone else. Really important ones, like where should my baby sleep? How am I going to feed my baby? And all the non-important day-to-day things too, like what are they going to wear today? Do they need a nappy change? Should I remove a layer? The weight of these decisions can feel heavy – especially so if you are tired (and let's face it, most of us are!).

The lack of free time, personal space and space to think can make it very hard to make a decision on how to tackle sleep, or indeed even whether or not you want to change anything. Sometimes we need to hit rock bottom to be mentally prepared to make a change or sometimes it might just be a gut feeling. Other times it takes the night from hell to make you stand up and realise enough is enough. It is so easy to revert to what you usually do – you might rock your baby to sleep and the thought of trying to do it any other way is terrifying. (There is nothing wrong with rocking your little one to sleep, by the way, but it is an example of something that can become unsustainable over time.) For one person it could be a really easy way to get their little one off to sleep, but for another it could become torture (and end up with a physio referral!). If you make the decision to change, it is important to be committed. It is important to align your views and your plan with your partner, or other caregivers in charge of your baby.

Having a clear plan, knowing what you are comfortable with and sticking to it feels hard, but it is what I want to help you do.

**SLOW AND STEADY . . .**

If your little one's sleep feels like a mammoth task, you should take a step backwards and look at it for what it is. It *is* something you can slowly improve, I promise. It is never too late: you are not a failure and your baby is not broken. Little steps day by day, creating new habits and trusting your instinct when you need to tweak your plan are key. Focus on daily improvements – the little wins – and take each day as it comes. Each day is a fresh learning opportunity for both you and your baby.

### No comparison

The parenting world is full of very passionate, intense and sometimes angry voices: angry at their own experiences; angry at the lack of support; angry that they feel let down by their support systems . . . You name it, I've heard it. I want to cut through that noise and explain, in simple terms, how to help your baby to sleep. I am not interested in how soon your neighbour's baby slept through the night or how long your sister's kids co-slept for. This is about *you*. You and *your* child.

Comparison really is the thief of joy and I want you to release yourself from this, right now.

Stop comparing your beautifully unique baby and unique set of circumstances to others around you.

## FEAR OF CRYING

I couldn't write this book without covering the topic of crying. When it comes to sleep, crying is an incredibly emotive topic. I truly believe that this is the number one barrier to working on sleep for most families. Crying can be uncomfortable, it can be triggering and it can leave us feeling helpless if we don't know what to do with it. You might have a baby who has been very vocal from birth or you might have a very relaxed baby who doesn't cry much. Either way, at some point your baby will have cried, and will continue to do so in the future.

We can't escape our baby's cry, nor should we want to. It is an unpleasant sound, designed by nature to get our attention as quickly as possible, and for important reasons. Our main job as a parent is to nurture our babies and to keep them safe, and to do this we need to know when they need us. We need to know if they are hungry, cold or need saving from a predator (think prehistoric babies!). Modern-day life is different now, but it's just as important to be in tune with our babies and their needs.

We should respond to crying, but our aim should never be to stop all crying or think that it's wrong for our children to ever be upset. Your child will never be happy 100 per cent of the time, and I think it is important for parents to be prepared for tears during babyhood and beyond – tears because they don't like their car seat, tears when you change their nappy, tears in the bath, tears because they don't like their dinner, tears because their first crush has broken their heart (you get where I'm going with this). We have a natural sense of urgency to stop crying, because it is our job, but also for other reasons. The first is because we have been made to believe that it's wrong – that if we are doing a good job, then our babies should be happy and not cry. This is a falsehood. It's totally unachievable and sets you up to fail.

It is possible to make changes with minimal tears, but it's

unlikely that there will be no tears at all. Most babies cry when we work on changing their usual way of doing things. We can, of course, change things in our little one's sleep environment, and possibly routine, without tears, but if they do cry you are not a terrible parent. Crying in itself is not dangerous and I promise you that if your baby cries, you are not a bad person or a bad parent. Many parents frantically try to stop their baby crying in public for fear of judgement from others. Maybe they need a feed, maybe they want to get out of their buggy, maybe they have a dirty nappy . . . Whatever the reason, of course we are going to respond to them as soon as we can, but we are made to feel that all eyes are on us and, rightly or wrongly, that other adults are judging our parenting. This taps into the myth of the 'good baby' – the baby who doesn't cry, who smiles at everyone, who sleeps through the night from the newborn weeks, who takes to food straight away, who doesn't touch dangerous things, who sits quietly as a toddler . . . there are no good or bad babies, and there are no good or bad parents.

If you visit our old friend the internet, you will find claims of 'no-cry' methods out there. I am afraid this is biologically impossible. Also, why would we want to avoid crying at all costs? We do not want to silence our babies. Their cry is often the only way they can communicate their needs to us. I want to know when my baby is wet, hungry, cold or needs me. Why do we need to stop the cry at every step? Is it because we ourselves feel uncomfortable with that crying? Crying in a loving home with a responsive parent is in no way damaging. Holding space for your little one's crying can be challenging, but it is often needed. When you move out of the newborn haze and your little one grows and becomes more interactive, you will find they communicate in many weird and wonderful ways. Truly listening to our babies is a lost art. We are far too busy looking at apps about what they 'should' be doing and listening to other people's opinions, when we are the ones who know our babies the best.

> You are your baby's expert.

## FEAR OF FAILURE

We all want to be the best parents that we can be so we can often feel shame around how our little ones sleep. You need to stop right now and forgive yourself for feeling rubbish about things. It is normal to have ups and downs with sleep. No baby and no parent is perfect.

In countless cases I have seen parents pleasantly surprised that improving sleep has been simple and far less painful than they anticipated. The thing is, you don't know until you try. Exploring the ideas in this book will hopefully release you from your fear of failure. Look at them as simply things you can try or things you can think about. Remember, there is no exam at the end of this. There is no test to pass. Whatever your outcome, you have not failed. With consistency, time and patience you'll find that you make progress. Whether it's a giant leap or tiny steps, it is progress, nonetheless.

## CREATING YOUR OWN RITUALS

Advocating on behalf of your baby and deciding what they really need is tough. But if anyone was made to do this for your child, it was you. Sleep is no different. You may find that when you start thinking about your own child's sleep you look back and reflect on your own experiences as a child. Those who had a strict upbringing might feel resistant to having a routine with their baby, or it could well go the other way and you crave the same stability. You might have fond memories of a particular teddy you took to bed and want to give that same opportunity for comfort to your child. You may feel nostalgic about certain bedtime stories and want to pass that on. Or you might have sad memories of an absent parent and a less happy home. Whatever this brings up for you, this is a fresh start, a chance to build healthy bedtime habits for you and your family that will be long-lasting. You can create your own bedtime rituals for your children to pass on to their children. Loving bedtime is a truly beautiful thing.

---

Loving your sleep space and being at peace where you sleep is a gift.

---

## NO RULES

Despite what many people will tell you there is no right or wrong – no 'rules' – when it comes to sleep. If you and your baby are happy in your sleep situation, you are all good. Opinions are everywhere – never forget that those who give you advice will be doing so from a position of bias. They are biased by their own experiences, their own childhoods, their own sleep struggles, and what worked or didn't work for their baby. Also, culturally and historically things have changed.

My nan used to put her children in their pram in the garden to sleep. This was commonplace in the post-war era. In many Eastern cultures it is the norm to co-sleep. In fact, you may find entire families in one room. I have had clients in the USA who have gone back to work full-time after six weeks' maternity leave and so have worked on shaping sleep religiously from an early age with this in mind. None of these things are wrong, and none are 'right' either. It's important to remember that, while the basic sleep science remains the same, our cultural and personal belief systems can vary wildly from family to family.

I have had many clients over the years who have come to me with their second, third, fourth or more babies. Although you may have more confidence in your decision-making, sleep doesn't necessarily come easier with each child you have. It really surprised me to find that each of my babies was so different. I naively assumed that we had a 'brand' of baby and that they would respond in the same way as each other. I couldn't have been more wrong. This is where having hard and fast rules around sleep isn't helpful. You need to take the reins and work out how to adapt what you are doing to your own baby. You friend's baby, your cousin's baby or whoever it is you are comparing yours to, may be very different to your own. That friend or cousin may also have an entirely different parenting style to you. And that's okay!

### All babies are different

*I once helped a family with five children. The parents were so embarrassed that they needed help with their fifth. He was the most 'difficult' baby they had had, but they felt like they should have 'known what they were doing' by now. I reassured them that this wasn't the case. This baby was an individual and their struggles were absolutely valid. It turns out that they had had some issues with infant reflux in the early days (as a result of positioning on the breast, which improved greatly with the help of a lactation consultant at around 12 weeks), but this meant that they had got into the habit of holding baby upright after feeds. The parents had been attending to their four other children at bedtime, so tended to wear the baby in a sling after his bedtime feed so that whoever was doing bedtime had their hands free.*

*This meant that he had never experienced falling asleep on his own at bedtime, and he would be held to sleep again during the night when he woke (several times). The family were certain that his reflux was 'fixed', but they were stuck in a rut with it. Their days were so busy, coordinating lives and rushing here, there and everywhere, that he was still held to sleep at 12 months – they just hadn't felt up to tackling it. The parents really wanted to move away from this, free up their evenings and have a more settled night. We worked on a plan together, and we reduced the night wakings to one, and then none by the end of our time together. It really was life-changing, and the parents went on to have baby number six the following year!*

## ADVICE FROM GRANDPARENTS

Advice will come from all areas, but it can be particularly tricky and sometimes awkward when it comes from grandparents . . .

1. Take a deep breath. Remember they probably mean well and that they love your baby, and you always have that in common.
2. Make sure they know and understand your boundaries. You might need to explain your rules on capping naps, on screen time, on sugar. It is okay to be firm. This isn't a reflection of what they did or do wrong, it's about how you want things to happen. This is your baby.
3. If on the odd occasion they care for your baby slightly differently, it's not the end of the world. If your little one stays up a little later with them or takes their nap in their buggy instead of their cot or goes a bit off their usual routine, it won't do any harm. It only becomes a problem if this is happening in their regular day-to-day lives, at the detriment to your baby's sleep. It may be slightly different if they are an actual carer for your baby on a regular basis because you are back at work – see Chapter 10.
4. If grandparents are turning up unannounced and you are finding that stressful, find some convenient times that would work, and communicate when you would like them to visit (for example, not during naptime!). Take the front foot and invite them when *you* want them to come.
5. Be a united front. If you have a partner, discuss the issues together before both communicating your wants/needs to your own parents or your in-laws.

## CHANGING YOUR MIND

One thing I want you to bear in mind is that it is always okay to change your mind. I think a lot of parents feel like they have chosen a particular path because it fits with their belief system, but people change and your needs fluctuate – go with your gut. If you choose one of the techniques in this book to work on your little one's sleep and it doesn't feel right, then change it up.

> It is always okay to change tack. In fact, doing so when you need to shows that you are in tune with your baby and the needs of your family.

It's not always easy to juggle it all and know what you need to do, but by giving you plenty of options I hope that you will choose the parts that feel right for you. I believe in 'pick 'n' mix parenting', which means you can take the bits you like and leave the rest. You don't ever have to label yourself as a particular type of parent. You don't have to choose between sleep and no sleep.

## YOU ARE THE BOSS

You know your baby better than anyone else out there. I want to help you tune into your baby's needs and give you some simple things you can try to get a more settled night's sleep. It's not always a straight road – there might be bumps along the way – but, you know what, that's okay too. Having the tools to fall back on when you hit those bumps can be really comforting. It's about navigating your little one's changing needs, while giving them the healthy foundations of a good night's sleep.

## KEY TAKEAWAYS

1. Always consider your individual needs and the needs of your family – what is sustainable for one parent may not be for another.
2. Sleep is everything, for our bodies and our minds.
3. Crying isn't necessarily a problem.
4. Sharing is key: a problem shared is a problem halved.
5. You can always change your mind – absolutely nothing is set in stone.

# PART 2

# 4

# GETTING THE BASICS RIGHT

Whenever I am working with a family on sleep, the first step is always to assess their baby's sleep environment. I want to help you create a sleep sanctuary for your baby and a place where you can make the most of your window of opportunity to sleep. When your baby is first born you will likely be getting less sleep than you are used to, so making sure the sleep that you do get is of a restorative quality is key.

Safer sleep guidance recommends keeping your baby in with you for the first six months of their life, so when we are thinking about sleep environment, in the early days at least, it will be your own bedroom.

It can be hard to navigate the wide range of baby sleep products on the market (just because it is sold in a shop doesn't mean that it is regulated or safe) and even choosing what your baby sleeps in can feel daunting. I'm going to give you some guidance in this chapter.

> Don't put pressure on yourself to create a picture-perfect nursery. Some people really love creating a beautiful nursery space before baby arrives, often inspired by those they see online, but you don't need to stress about it if it's

not something you are ready for or have the space or funds for. Keep in mind that your baby just needs you and somewhere safe to sleep.

## WHAT SHOULD YOUR BABY SLEEP IN?

Your baby will need a clean, safe space to sleep in. You could choose a Moses basket or crib (bedside cribs are popular), or you might choose to use a cot from the outset. A lot will depend on the space you have available. You will need a firm, flat mattress, preferably new for each baby as there is some research that shows using a mattress from outside the home can increase the risk of sudden infant death syndrome (SIDS – the sudden, unexpected and unexplained death of an apparently healthy baby). If you are using a second-hand mattress, The Lullaby Trust (see page 284) advises ensuring it was previously protected by a waterproof cover, and that it is in good condition, with no rips or tears. It should still be firm and flat and properly fit the Moses basket, crib or cot you are using.

### Moses basket

In the early weeks especially, it is likely you will have your baby sleeping in the same room as you in the evenings and the daytime. This is when a Moses basket can come in handy as it is so portable. (A carrycot works too, so long as it has a firm, flat and waterproof mattress.) Please note that your baby shouldn't sleep in a buggy, bouncer or car seat – if they fall asleep in any of these, move them to their Moses basket, crib or cot.

### Bedside crib

A bedside crib attaches to the side of your bed and your baby will be able to sleep in it up to six months, unlike a Moses basket which they are likely to outgrow sooner. It is a good option if you don't have space for a full-size cot in your bedroom and also if you are breastfeeding, as it gives you quick access to your baby at night without you having to get out of bed. This can be particularly helpful if you have had a caesarean section. The disadvantage of a bedside crib is that it isn't portable, like a Moses basket, so you will need to supervise your baby's naps at home in your bedroom up to the age of six months.

### Straight to cot

Using a cot from newborn is the most cost-effective solution, as it means buying only one item for your baby to sleep in, which will last well into toddlerhood. The downside is the size – not everyone has the space for a full-size cot in their bedroom. It is also not at all portable so you will need to supervise naps in your bedroom until your baby is six months old. It can also feel strange to see a tiny baby in a huge space, but be reassured they will be absolutely fine. Most cots have adjustable mattress heights too, which are easier on your back when you're putting your baby down for sleep. Make sure they are dressed appropriately so that they don't get cold. Don't be tempted to use a sleep nest (see page 59) in the cot as these do not adhere to safer sleep guidance. For safe sleeping, it is always best to have a cot clear of other items.

---

**SAFE SLEEP**

Knowing that you have followed all the safety guidelines will allow you to relax more and help you to get a better night's sleep.

- You should always put your baby down to sleep on their back (not on their side or front), with a clear cot, crib or Moses basket free of loose bedding or toys.

- Make sure your baby's feet are at the foot of their sleep space so that they can't wriggle down under their bedding – known as the 'feet-to-foot' position.
- Sheets and blankets should be firmly tucked in to shoulder height only or use a baby sleeping bag (see page 56).
- Duvets and pillows should be avoided until your baby is at least a year old, and their head should always be uncovered.
- You should not share a bed with your baby under any of the following conditions: they were born prematurely or at a low birth weight, you've consumed alcohol or drugs, you smoke, or you're excessively tired. (See page 170 for more on bed-sharing.)

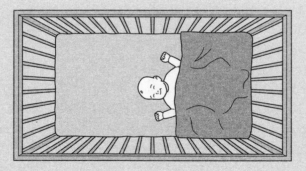

*To prevent your baby wriggling down under the covers, place them in the 'feet-to-foot' position. This means their feet are at the end of the crib, cot or Moses basket.*

Once your baby can roll both ways, it is important to allow them to find their own comfortable sleeping position. While they are learning to do this, lots of supervised tummy time during the day can help them to develop this skill (see page 112).

## BED-SHARING

In this book I will use the term 'bed-sharing' to mean sharing a bed with your baby and 'co-sleeping' to mean sleeping near to your baby (for example, in the same room, with your baby in a crib or cot). The terms are often used interchangeably, but I will use 'bed-sharing' here to be clear about what I mean. It is normal for your baby to want to be close to you, so some families struggle to get their baby into their own sleep space. If you wish to bed-share, or end up doing this out of necessity, then you can make an informed choice to do so. Some families find they get more sleep if they bed-share, while others don't sleep a wink. If it does work for you, the important thing is that you do it safely. Never fall asleep with your baby on a sofa or in an armchair. This increases their chance of SIDS by 50 times. If you feel like you are going to fall asleep while feeding your baby, it is much safer to feed them in your bed where you can lie on your side.

I want to be honest and practical about bed-sharing. So many people bed-share but are ashamed to admit it, so end up doing it unsafely. Although a baby's own sleep space is the safest place for them to be, I would really like to remove the stigma around bed-sharing. Some people actively choose to do it and some do it out of necessity, as they can't see any other viable alternative (this is where my methods will come in later, if you want a plan for stopping – see Chapter 8).

These are the guidelines from The Lullaby Trust about bed-sharing:

1. Keep all adult bedding clear of your baby. This includes duvets and pillows, or anything else that could cause your baby to overheat or that could obstruct their breathing. I always recommend a clear bed. Baby should have their own appropriately fitting sleeping bag – this removes the danger

of loose bedding. (If you are bed-sharing, you can't tuck a blanket in with their feet at the foot of the bed.) Some parents find that they get cold without a duvet covering them entirely – so wearing a warm hoodie can be a quick fix to this! A zipped one is good if you are breastfeeding.

2. You should always put baby to sleep on their back, even if they are next to you. If they fall asleep nursing, you should roll them onto their backs. Nursing your baby in a side-lying position can be good for this, and once they come off, you can roll them onto their back.

3. You should keep all other children and pets out of the bed.

4. Be mindful of where in your bed your baby is placed – make sure they won't fall out of the bed or get wedged between the wall and the bed.

5. If you or your partner smoke, drink alcohol or take drugs (including medications that make you drowsy) you should never bed-share.

6. If your baby was premature (born before 37 weeks) or weighs 2.5 kilograms or less it isn't safe to bed-share.

See The Lullaby Trust (see page 284) for more information on safer sleeping.

### Time for a change

*I met baby Anna and her parents when she was eight months old. She had slept in her mum's bed from birth as her mum found it much easier to breastfeed this way and got more sleep than trying to transfer her into her crib. Dad was sleeping in the spare room. Anna's parents decided it was time for a change – they wanted her to sleep in her own sleep space, and potentially her own room. Mum had enjoyed bed-sharing up until now, but Anna had started wriggling and crawling under the* duvet which didn't feel safe or relaxing anymore. She had also started to wake more frequently and was getting very frustrated at the breast during night wakings. She had gone from waking a couple of times at night to six to eight times. Mum was breastfeeding each time, but this had become unsustainable and was making Mum miserable.

Anna's mum didn't want to do controlled crying as she was worried that it would be too much change at once. The parents decided to stay in the room with Anna while she settled. They considered a slower transition from bed-sharing, but decided to just go for it and see how she got on. We made sure she had a great routine and that she was really ready for bedtime (her last nap finished by 3pm in order for her to be sleepy and tired for a 7pm bedtime). There were some tears, but they were always accompanied – Mum and Dad took turns to pat her and comfort her verbally. She cried for a total of 15 minutes. This was with either Mum or Dad present. They were careful to leave as soon as she was calm. She woke three times on the first night and only once on the second night – at each of these wakings she cried for between three and fifteen minutes. On the third night she slept through.

The change in Anna's sleep also had a positive impact on her naps. For the first time since she was a newborn, she took a two-hour lunchtime nap. Her parents discovered that it was best to cap her morning nap to 30 minutes. Previously they had been allowing her a long morning nap, which was a catch-up from her broken nights. She would then refuse a second nap until late afternoon, causing settling problems at bedtime. Previously she wouldn't settle until 9pm on some nights.

Dad was pleased to return to the marital bed. Mum said she felt quite guilty about letting go of bed-sharing, but it wasn't serving her anymore. It turns out that they were all much happier with their new set-up. When I finished up with them, Anna was going to bed at 7.15pm and mainly sleeping through until 6.30/7am.

## BEDDING

You will need well-fitting sheets for the cot, crib or Moses basket. I would suggest investing in a few as it's quite common for your little one to posset (bring up milk after a feed) in their sleep space. Some babies are more 'sicky' than others.

### Sleeping bags

Sleeping bags are really great option for babies to sleep in as they can't kick them off or get tangled up in them. You know that your baby won't wake up cold because they have kicked their blanket off, and you won't wake up panicking that they have pulled their blanket up over their face. Sleeping bags are also a great signal as part of your bedtime routine, so that your baby knows sleep is on the way. I tend to use them for naptimes too (although you don't have to), to keep the consistent message that sleep time is coming. Make sure your baby is wearing appropriate clothing so they don't overheat and that you are using a weight-appropriate bag; check the tog for the time of year and the temperature of your room. There should be a guide on the label.

> For very young babies, depending on their size and weight, you might find that a cellular blanket tucked in around baby (below shoulder level) is a better option. Always follow safe sleeping guidelines (see box on page 51).

## SWADDLING

You might have seen pictures of babies wrapped up like little burritos – these are babies who have been swaddled in a blanket. If you give birth in hospital, it is likely that your midwife will help you swaddle your baby for the first time. Swaddling is commonplace with newborns as it mimics the security of the womb, helping them to feel safe, and helps with the 'Moro reflex', the startle reflex that causes them to wake themselves up with their flailing arms. Not all babies like being swaddled and it isn't essential, so I encourage you to think of it as a tool in your parenting toolbox. Perhaps try it to see how your baby responds. For some families it can be an absolute game changer, while for others it's unnecessary and the baby sleeps fine without it.

Below is step-by-step guidance on how to swaddle your baby. For guidance on how to gradually stop swaddling your baby, see page 124.

1. Always follow safe sleeping guidance and put a swaddled baby to sleep on their back, never on their front or side.
2. You shouldn't swaddle your baby if you are bed-sharing.
3. If your baby is showing any signs of rolling you should stop swaddling immediately (see page 124 for guidance on how to stop swaddling). To be on the safe side, I advise stopping swaddling by 16 weeks at the latest. I also think it is helpful for babies to have access to their hands for settling purposes. Some babies suck their thumb, fingers or hands to soothe. This is helpful for sleep! For this reason, I don't use mittens to cover hands (the exception being if your little one suffers from eczema).
4. Always use a light material. Thin cotton or muslin is ideal. Never use a fleece material – I have seen fleece swaddle blankets, but these are not safe due to potential overheating. Don't put any extra blankets over your swaddled baby.
5. Make sure their head is always uncovered.
6. Don't swaddle baby if they are poorly and have a fever.
7. Always check in on your baby and make sure they are not too hot – check the back of their neck and remove some bedclothes if the baby's skin is hot and sweaty.

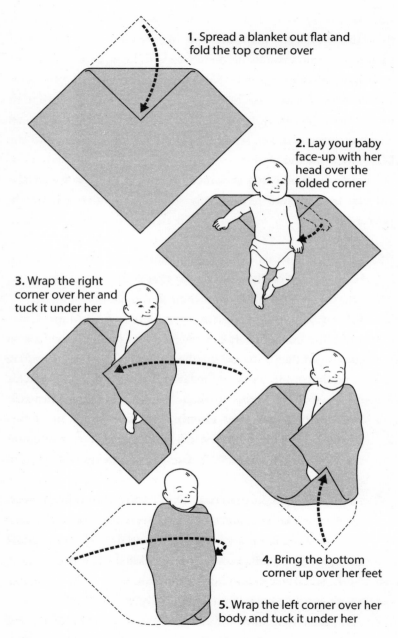

1. Spread a blanket out flat and fold the top corner over

2. Lay your baby face-up with her head over the folded corner

3. Wrap the right corner over her and tuck it under her

4. Bring the bottom corner up over her feet

5. Wrap the left corner over her body and tuck it under her

*Step-by-step swaddling instructions*

8. Make sure your swaddle is secure – you don't want it to be too loose and potentially cover your baby's face.

9. Be careful around your baby's hips – the swaddle should be tight enough to be sure it won't ride up, but if it is too tight on the hips it can cause problems. Your baby's hips should be in a slight flexion when you swaddle them (this means not completely straight).

10. There are some good 'easy swaddle' products on the market, so if you choose one of these make sure it is a breathable fabric, fits well and meets safety standards. These can be really useful if you get flustered and are struggling with a traditional swaddle.

## BABY POSITIONERS

You might have seen the popular sleeping pods (sometimes called nests), which influencers and celebs place into their baby's cot or crib, alongside other products such as fancy pillows. They are often really pretty and form part of the 'picture-perfect' nurseries you will see on social media, but they are not safe and go against safe sleeping guidelines (see box on page 51). Hammocks are sometimes marketed as an alternative to a cot or there are some that you put over a cot. Neither are tested or approved for infant sleep.

You will also see pillows being sold that are targeted towards parents whose babies have flat head syndrome (whereby prolonged periods of lying on their back causes a baby to develop a flattened head) – these should only be used under the advice of your healthcare practitioner. There are other things you can do – like seeing a paediatric physio, osteopath or chiropractor, and encouraging lots of tummy time during the day (see page 112).

It is really common for newborns to want to be enclosed and held tight, so I can see why these products have become popular. However, as babies grow, I truly believe they need the space to move around. As your baby's sleep matures, some of these products can actually hinder sleep – they stop your baby moving during their sleep, which is a really normal part of their development.

---

You want your baby to be comfortable in their own sleep space without props and have the freedom to move and practise their motor skills.

---

Anything that fixes baby in position or wedges them in can pose a risk. We know that baby sleeping on anything but a firm, flat, clean mattress, or having loose bedding, can increase the risk of SIDS. There is a chance of overheating and the possibility of obstructed airways. We shouldn't put baby to sleep among any raised or cushioned areas. This also means that cot bumpers are not safe. They pose the same risk as positioners, but with the added risk that babies could become trapped between the bumper and the side of their cot. I have also heard of older babies using them like a ladder to climb out of their cots – also not safe!

The best thing you can do is save your money and invest time in working on your little one's sleep in a safe way with the practices I'll discuss later in this book.

## ROOM-SHARING FOR THE FIRST SIX MONTHS

We know from the latest research that sharing a room with your baby for the first six months of their lives significantly reduces the risk of SIDS. The safest place for them to sleep is in the same room as their parents.

So, what it is about sharing a room which keeps our babies safe? We are still unsure of the exact reasons why, but what we do know is that studies have found fewer babies die from SIDS when they are in the room with their parents as opposed to sleeping alone. I think we can assume that one of the possible reasons is that we might respond quicker to our babies and notice if they are in difficulty. Room-sharing can make breastfeeding easier, which is also a protector against SIDS.

Thankfully, since the 1990s and the 'back to sleep campaign' (the introduction of the advice to put babies to sleep on their backs), SIDS has become far rarer.

I want to reassure you that there is no rule that once your baby turns six months you must move them out of your room. You can do this later if you prefer, there really is no rush. See page 137 for advice on moving your baby into their own room.

---

It's all about making an informed choice and working out what is best for you and your family.

---

## BABY MONITORS

While your baby is sharing a room with you or you are supervising their sleep, you don't really need a monitor. Once they are old enough to sleep independently, you will need to be able to check in on them. It can also be useful when you are working on sleep to keep an eye on them. Here are some things to consider when you are looking for a monitor:

1. How big is your home and what is the range on the monitor?
2. Depending on your budget, there are video or just audio monitors.
3. Some monitors will be able to tell you the temperature of the room, which can be a useful feature.

4.  Some can be used with a smartphone or laptop so you can monitor baby if you are away or at work and someone else is looking after them.

5.  Some have lullabies or white noise (see page 68) as a feature on them.

6.  There are some on the market that have sensors and heart rate monitors. While there is no evidence that these are protective against SIDS, they can give parents added peace of mind that the alarm would go off if their baby stopped breathing. Still, they shouldn't be relied on solely and babies should still sleep in the same room as their parents for the first six months.

If you don't have a spare room, be reassured that many families across the world continue to room-share with their children either through choice or necessity for years. You could make the corner of your room a little 'baby space' or use a room divider if you find you disturb your little one or vice versa. You can get some beautiful dividers. Equally your room might just look like it always has, with a cot in it. As always, do whatever works for you.

## SLEEP TRAINING WHILE ROOM-SHARING

I am often asked if you can 'sleep train' (see Chapter 8) while room-sharing. The answer is yes, absolutely. Sharing a room doesn't mean you have to put up with disturbed sleep for years. You just need to be strategic about the method that you use. You can choose any of the methods detailed in this book (see Chapter 8), but if you choose one where you are exiting the room, you may need to temporarily camp out in your front room or be prepared to be in and out of bed while you implement your changes.

### Sharing with a sibling

Ideally, if you want to try this or need to because of a lack of space, both baby and child will be sleeping well before you make the change. You can think about staggering bedtimes according to their sleep needs. Explaining to your older child what is going on is important. Sharing a room can bring comfort and security, so don't be afraid to do it. They will likely disturb each other a lot less than you expect.

## TWINS AND TRIPLETS

You can put twins together in a single cot while they are small enough (this is called co-bedding), but you can't do this with a Moses basket, which is too small. Multiples are used to being close to one another and being together will help them regulate body temperature and feel safe. All the same safe sleeping guidance applies, though – put them on their backs to sleep and position them with their feet at opposite ends of the cot, with the tops of their heads facing one another. This way they can both have their feet at the foot of the cot. Alternatively, if they are still small enough, they can go side by side in the cot, with their feet at the foot.

Triplets can lie side by side across a cot, with their feet at the side. As your multiples grow, you can put them in separate cots or cribs close to one another. Once they can roll, you should put them in separate cots as it becomes a safety issue if they were to obstruct their sibling's airways. If they start to disturb one another as they get older, you can put them in separate rooms if you prefer (and have the space!). Bear in mind they still need to share a room with a parent until the age of six months.

A key piece of kit I recommend for multiples is a bouncer. This means you can be settling a baby in their cot or crib, while bouncing the other baby with your foot (before transferring them to their crib, as bouncers are not a safe place for them to sleep). This works well with younger babies. You can, of course, have both babies in their crib and take turns with the settling (if they need it).

## TEMPERATURE

Have you ever sat on the sofa in the evening and suddenly felt chilly? It is likely your body telling you to go to bed! As humans, we all sleep a little better when it is on the cool side. Our body temperature starts to fall as we approach bedtime, so having a nice cool room can work with this. The most comfortable, and safe, temperature for you or your baby's room is 16–20°C – you might want to invest in a room thermometer. While we should adhere to this whenever possible, sometimes it is just out of our control – when we have a heatwave or a very cold snap for example.

Each baby is different so it's important to check in on your baby and their temperature. It is normal for their hands and feet to feel cold (see box below). The best way to check your baby's temperature is to feel their chest or the back of their neck. If they feel hot or sweaty you should remove a layer. Bear in mind that they should never sleep with a hat on indoors (so remove it when you come in from a walk), and babies who are unwell often need fewer layers. Always remember to remove the rain cover if you come in from a walk and your baby has fallen asleep in their pram – or, ideally, move them to a crib or cot for better airflow. It is important that babies don't overheat, especially when they are sleeping.

In hot weather, you can use a fan but be careful not to point it directly at baby, and it should be out of reach. Babies can't control their body temperature like we can, so although it might be hot they can still get a chill. Safer sleep guidance suggests a fan can be beneficial to keep the room cool, and therefore protective against SIDS, but we should be mindful of positioning.

Your baby may get a temperature irrespective of their environment, if their body is fighting an infection or a virus. If you are ever concerned about your baby's temperature, always consult your doctor.

## COLD HANDS AND FEET

It is normal for young babies to have cold extremities. Firstly, they don't move around very much so they have less blood flow to their limbs. They have an immature blood circulation system under the age of three months, so, as the blood flows around the body, less goes to their hands and feet, and more goes to the important bits – the heart and the busy digestive system (think of all those feeds!).

### In cold winter months

In the colder months, be mindful of layers. You want your baby to be warm so dress them appropriately for cold weather, but ensure they do not overheat. When you are returning home from the outside, make sure you remove all their outdoor clothing, even if they are sleeping.

1. Ideally their bedclothes should still be breathable cotton; try not to use fleece or synthetic materials.
2. You might want to turn your heating off at night or keep it at a steady temperature. Don't be tempted to turn it up very high in the evenings, when your baby might overheat if they are already asleep and you are in another room. If you tend to turn your heating off overnight, be mindful that baby might feel chilly in the early hours when the temperature tends to drop. You could put the heating on a timer to come on so it is warm by the time you all get up.
3. Do not put a hat on your baby at night.

### In hot summer months

1. When out and about with your baby, keep them in the shade as much as possible. Cross to the shady side of the street and keep them out of the sun, especially between 11am and 3pm when it is at its hottest. You can apply sunscreen to babies over six months, and always put a sun hat on them and dress them in loose, light clothing.
2. Never cover prams, buggies or car seats with muslins or blankets. This heats them up like a greenhouse. A parasol is ideal, or a safety-checked cover designed for this purpose will also work. In the car, it is better to get a shade that attaches to the window.
3. If you have a garden, a little paddling pool in the shade is lovely and your baby will enjoy splashing. (But remember to never leave any child unattended near water.) Ideally have the water at a moderate temperature. Cool is good, but if it's too cold your baby won't like it.
4. Close the curtains during the day to keep the sun out – it can feel counter-intuitive, but wall insulation can keep heat out, as

well as in. You can then reopen the windows when baby goes to bed to let some airflow in.

5. You can try putting bottles of frozen water in front of a fan (which serves as a mini air con solution!). You can also hang a wet towel over a chair or door – pre-freezing this helps. The evaporating water cools the air. If using a fan, place it well away from baby so that they cannot grab it and do not have it blowing directly on to them.

6. If it is very hot in your baby's room, they can just sleep in a vest or nappy. There are very thin sleeping bags on the market (0.5 tog) if they need to sleep with something on them.

7. Airflow in your baby's room trumps blackout! It's much more important that they don't overheat, so in extreme temperatures don't close their door, to allow air through.

8. Lukewarm baths before bed are good. Make sure they aren't too cold, as that will boost circulation (your body's way of keeping warm). When we go to sleep at night our body temperature needs to drop to go to sleep (this will happen naturally). Having a bath before bed helps – as the water evaporates from our skin it cools us down.

9. Place a cold (not frozen) flannel on the baby's forehead to cool them a little if they are struggling. (Never leave them like this unattended, though.)

10. A cotton muslin between you when feeding or cuddling can help with the sweating!

11. If you live in a house and it is too hot upstairs, don't be afraid to do naps downstairs. If your home is very hot it could even be worth a trip to a local air-conned cafe or supermarket for naptime!

12. If your home is too hot at bedtime, you can surrender your evening. Take a picnic to the park and sit under some trees – it could be a romantic change of routine.

In hot temperatures your baby might want to feed more than usual, so go with it. If you are formula feeding you can offer a little cooled boiled water between their usual feeds. Breastfed babies don't need water until they are eating solid foods – your breast milk adapts during hot weather to quench their thirst.

If you are working on improving your baby's sleep, I would consider pausing until the heatwave has passed. Extreme temperatures can be tricky to get to sleep in, and to stay asleep, so return to your sleep work when it's a bit cooler.

## WHITE NOISE

White noise is a combination of frequencies that sounds like static or like a washing machine, raindrops or a fan. These gentle, rhythmic sounds all work in the same way, helping to calm your baby and therefore helping them to sleep. A baby has been used to the calming sound of a heartbeat in the womb and the sound of blood whooshing through the placenta. Not only can white noise be useful to help calm baby, it can also drown out any sudden noises which may startle them – a dog barking, a lively sibling or the postman knocking at the door, for example. (I highly recommend putting a sign on the door when baby is sleeping – I learned this the hard way myself!)

White noise should be fairly quiet – if you are unsure then I always say no louder than the sound of a running shower. If you are ever unsure, err on the side of caution with volume. Neonatal intensive care units are limited to 50 decibels, so bear this in mind.

White noise should be kept on continuously through the night or for the duration of naps if you are using it. If your baby stirs, we want the white noise to be available to them, as it was when they fell asleep in the first place. It is important to keep things as consistent as possible overnight.

Pink noise has become more popular in recent years. This is white noise but with reduced higher frequencies. There are claims that it is more soothing than white noise and will help your baby fall into a deeper sleep for longer. There isn't a great deal of research on this, so the jury is out as to which type of noise is most effective, but for the reason that it may prematurely encourage deeper sleep I would only try it if your baby is over the age of six months.[1]

White noise is definitely not an essential for all babies, it's just something you can try if you like and see if your baby benefits from it. You can stop using it whenever you want – just gradually turn down the volume across the course of a few days, and if there is no difference in your baby's sleep you can just switch it off.

Bear in mind that if you choose to use white noise, you will have to listen to it too!

Personally, it isn't something I used with my babies – mainly because I didn't want to listen to it myself. We are all different, so it's about what works for your baby, and for you.

## SLEEPING ON THE GO

Your baby will fall asleep on the go at some point. After all, they have been in the womb for nine months being rocked to sleep, so it is very natural for them to nap this way. They might fall asleep in their pram/buggy, car seat, baby carrier or baby swing and these can be good options for helping them to fall asleep if naps in the cot or Moses basket aren't going well.

However, baby swings, bouncers and car seats are not safe spaces for your baby to *continue* to sleep and they should always be transferred to a firm, flat mattress. If you find that your baby always wakes on transfer, it would be advisable to work on settling them in a cot or crib in the first place.

There are, of course, some babies who buck the trend and won't sleep anywhere other than their cot or crib. This is okay, and please don't worry. It just means you'll need to do a bit of planning around naps. Try to let it go and relax if they don't sleep when you are out on the odd occasion. As baby grows and takes fewer naps, this will feel easier to navigate.

### Sleeping in the car

If small babies travel in an upright position for too long, they may be at risk of breathing difficulties. They should be in a car for no longer than two hours at a time and should have regular breaks. An adult should sit with baby if possible or supervise with a baby car mirror. Remember also that babies should travel in rearward-facing baby seats, which provide better protection for their head, neck and spine in the case of a collision. If they slump forward in their seat, you should stop and change their position. Your baby shouldn't wear a coat or a snowsuit in the car – this stops the safety harness from working as it should as the extra layer acts as a barrier so the harness isn't as close to their body as it needs to be. Removing hats and outdoor clothing also prevents overheating, which we also need to be mindful of.

I have had many clients over the years who have resorted to driving their baby around for hours trying to get them to sleep, and not stopping for fear of their baby waking up. This is unsustainable – and inadvisable for the reasons I've stated above. Break the habit and work on a more practical and healthy way to get your baby to sleep (see Chapter 8).

### Sleeping in the pram or buggy

This is, of course, fine for daytime naps as long as the baby is lying flat. In fact, I highly recommend some naps to be taken outside on the go – it can be good for you both to get out. Make sure your baby is wearing appropriate layers for the temperature so they are not too hot or too cold. Don't cover the pram with blankets to darken them or protect them from the sun – only use a cover that is designed for this purpose and safety-tested (see page 66).

### Using a baby carrier

Sleeping in a baby carrier is also fine (and very useful so you can be hands free!), just be careful to follow the baby sling safety rules. Remember the acronym T.I.C.K.S, created by the UK Sling Consortium:[2]

- Tight
- In view at all times
- Close enough to kiss
- Keep chin off chest
- Supported back

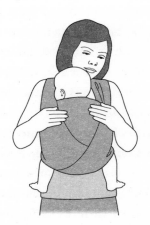

*Safest position for baby wearing*

You want baby nice and close, and in view so you can see their face. Baby should be close to your chin and close enough to kiss and they should never be curled so that their chin is on their chest. Their back should also be supported in a natural position. All these things keep your baby from slumping and restricting their airways, and keeps them safe.

If you have very recently given birth, make sure you don't overdo it carrying baby. I would advise working on your pelvic floor and core strength before carrying your baby for an extended period. This is especially important if you have had a C-section, suffered any tearing or trauma to your pelvic floor, or are recovering from pelvic girdle pain.

## DARKNESS

There is not a rule that you must have your room pitch black, but the fact is that darkness helps humans sleep. We used to fall asleep not long after the sun went down and wake up at sunrise – obviously this is not the case in modern life, but our biology hasn't changed. Our sleep is ruled by our circadian rhythm, and one of the things that can influence this is darkness and light. For the purposes of our babies, it is useful to have a darkened room at bedtime, when during the summer months it may well still be light outside. It can also help with early risers (and will help you get back to sleep if you are doing a feed in the early hours and the sun is rising).

Naptimes don't need to be in darkness, but if you find your baby struggles to switch off you can reassess it. Newborns tend to be quite happy sleeping in a light room, but if they are finding it difficult you can try drawing the curtains. As your baby grows and becomes more aware of their environment you may find they need some darkness to combat their FOMO (fear of missing out!), which tends to happen at around three to four months old (see page 76). Investing in some blackout blinds or curtains may just change your life if you have a baby who is hard to settle.

It is good to expose your baby to lots of light during the day, and to keep things nice and dark at night-time. This is how they learn to differentiate day from night, and how their circadian rhythm develops. If you ensure enough exposure to daylight across the day, you can do whatever you like for naps. Your baby won't get confused between night and day as long as they are not napping for too long during the day. If you are feeding your baby responsively, and enough, during the day and exposing them to natural light then they will grow to understand the difference between day and night. We never want babies to sleep through a feed, and we should be getting out and about at least once a day where possible (more on this later!) to get some fresh air and natural light. We also need to think practically – if you have other children, or need to run errands, or even just want to get out of the home for your mental health, it is always okay to do naps out and about.

The best product I can recommend for night-times is an amber reading light. I discovered this when I was searching for a sleep-friendly coloured light for my second baby. The best colour for sleep is amber, red, pink or orange. They don't 'help' us sleep, but they don't hinder it like blue or white light. So, I found an inexpensive amber clip-on reading light that changed my life. It meant that I could do nappy changes and night feeds in the dark without disturbing our sleep. It helped me get back to sleep quicker too. There is nothing worse than lying there for hours awake after a feed when your baby has nodded off. This light is often sold out thanks to me mentioning it to everyone who ever asks me for a recommendation!

I hope that this chapter has given you the confidence to set up your sleep space, knowing it is safe for your baby. Next, we are going to talk about the early days of sleep, the practicalities of what to do with your baby and how to protect your own sleep and get adequate rest.

# 5

# THE FOURTH
# TRIMESTER

The first few months of your baby's life are often referred to as the 'fourth trimester' because they are almost like an extension of the time in the womb. It is a period of huge physical and emotional change for both your baby and you as parents. They are adjusting to being in the world and you are adjusting to your new roles – both in a physical capacity, as well as mentally and emotionally.

Lots of people will tell you to simply go with the flow at this stage and that it's all just about getting through it. While I agree that this might be right for some people, others may be keen to find some solid, tangible advice they can put in place to start gently shaping their little one's sleep. This might also be vital for the parents' physical and mental health.

The key is to go gently on yourself and your baby. Don't put too much pressure on 'achieving' solid sleep. Those first few weeks can feel like you are treading water, just trying to keep your head up, or they might fly by in a haze. Some families start to emerge from this and find they have fallen into a bit more of a pattern with their days. Others may have hit a wall of sleep deprivation and decide they want to have a bit more structure. Whichever way you feel, it is totally valid. I will say throughout this book that the feelings you have about your little one's sleep are okay, whatever they are, and your journey with your baby might look different to your friends' and family's babies, or different to what you thought yours would look like.

## A TIME OF ADJUSTMENT

The first few weeks of your baby's life can be a real shock to the system for everyone. You may never have experienced sleep deprivation like this before, or you may have a baby who sleeps a fair bit. The key thing is finding your coping mechanisms and learning how to advocate for yourself, your baby and your family, which means seeking support when you need it and holding your boundaries when you don't want outside input. You are getting to know your baby, which takes time. You will get to know their own individual cues, their personalities, their first smile. It will get easier, and more sleep is going to become available, I promise. I am going to help you to make the most of these windows of opportunity to help you and your baby to get a bit more rest.

Many parents will wonder if they will ever sleep again, and it might not feel like it in those early days, but I promise that you will. This is just a fleeting moment in time, even if it doesn't feel that way right now. Each week of your baby's life is full of rapid change and development, but they are still really teeny. These first few months are about finding your rhythm, getting to know your baby and capitalising on the sleep that you do get. We want to give you and your family the best chance at getting a good night's sleep, even if that means it is broken up with night feeds. It isn't true when people say you must just wait it out either – we do have the chance in these first few months to lay some great foundations for solid sleep later on. Once we pass the first few weeks of adjustment, some babies are ready for a bit more of a rhythm to their days and their nights.

The key thing is finding your coping mechanisms and learning how to advocate for yourself, your baby and your family.

### Gradual change

As your baby grows in these first few months, they will gradually begin to need less sleep overall, go longer between naps and (hopefully!) sleep more at night. They will start to become more physically active during the day, alert and less likely to nod off so regularly. Generally, most newborns find it very easy to sleep, whatever their environment (there are always exceptions to this, especially those babies who have a difficult start to life). Overall, daylight doesn't stop newborns from napping during the day, and neither does noise. However, as they grow this may well change! You might also see some loose patterns appearing, and you might find it easier to start to structure your day a little (if that's something you want to do). I am a big fan of a 'loose' structure even with small babies. It is unlikely that your baby will 'sleep through the night' at this stage (unless you are really lucky!), but we can absolutely start working on optimising sleep for you and your family.

## THE FIRST 24 HOURS

So, let's start at the very beginning. Whether you had your little one at hospital or at home, that moment when you are left alone with your bundle of joy can feel a little overwhelming to say the least. It is normal to be totally in love and in a bubble (or not quite yet), and at the same time wonder what on earth you are supposed to do with your baby. It is normal to have mixed emotions, to feel overwhelmed, excited and a whole host of other feelings. All reactions are valid, honestly. Don't feel like you are feeling the wrong way – it can also take time to bond with your baby.

There is no wrong way to feel after you have just carried
and birthed another human.

You may or may not feel like you are in shock. You may or may not feel like you are on cloud nine. You may not really know what's going on. Every reaction and experience is different, and every feeling is valid.

Whatever your birth experience, it is likely that you will be feeling tired. The irony of the situation is that your body has gone through an immense change – it has birthed a life and is trying to heal. Of all the times in your life this is probably when you need to sleep the most. This is also the time when you are responsible for looking after another small person who is entirely dependent on you and who wakes at (very!) regular intervals for feeds, changes and cuddles. It is hard. I am not going to sugar-coat it. Some of you might have had long inductions and multiple nights of sleep deprivation before you even got to this point. Some of you may have had pregnancy insomnia; some may have had major surgery. Let's just say, you are going to need to rest wherever possible. You will hear me talking about prioritising your rest and your window of opportunity for sleep in other parts of this book. Basically, if you get a chance to rest, make sure you give it a shot.

## Your baby's world

Your baby will be totally unfamiliar with the world they have come into, which will be a bit of a shock to them. Until now, they have been cocooned in a warm, dark, comfortable place with food on tap via the placenta. They have never known hunger, never known clothing, never known what it is like to be separated from you. For all these reasons, your baby is likely to be very sleepy in the first 24 hours.

They will have their first ever feed – which takes a lot of energy for them to do whether it is breast or bottle. It's new for them to need to wake and ask to be fed, and it's new for them to learn how to suckle from a breast or bottle. It is quite common that you might need to wake them to feed.

### Skin-to-skin contact

I am a big fan of as much skin-to-skin as possible as soon as your baby is born. It is never too late to do this (in fact I highly recommend it for older babies too if they are upset). Not everyone has the fairy tale birth where they hold baby immediately, so it's a case of as soon as you are able (and if you are not able then your birth partner can do this). Not only does skin-to-skin help you bond with your baby, but it will help stimulate your milk supply if you are breastfeeding, will relax you after your birth experience and can help to regulate your baby's heartrate and breathing, and reduce your stress levels if you are in pain. Generally, less stress from both parent and baby will more likely result in better sleep (when you do get the opportunity).

If we are in 'fight or flight' mode after birth it can be hard to switch off and get any rest. The 'fight or flight' mode is a response from the body to a perceived threat, danger or stress. It is there to protect us and to make sure we could run away from danger (a bear that might eat us, for example!) or to fight. It means we are full of adrenalin, which cleverly keeps us going, but we need that to start to reduce if we are to rest and recover. Even ten minutes of skin-to-skin can reduce the stress hormone cortisol and help the production of oxytocin, the love hormone that makes us feel happy and relaxed.

For those parents who have used a surrogate or adopted a baby, these feelings, experiences and the transformation into a new parent are no less valid or potentially difficult. Skin-to-skin contact is important for everyone – biological parent, birth parent or however our babies enter this world.

## THE SECOND NIGHT

I want to prepare you for something that, although hard, can be easier to handle if you are expecting it – the second night with your baby. This is sometimes referred to as 'second night syndrome'. It isn't really spoken about enough in my opinion and, if we could be a little more prepared for this, I think parents would be less likely to freak out and think that something is wrong with their baby (although you should always trust your gut in this respect).

The theory is that your baby is really tired from being born. It's a pretty stressful process for them, however they come out. By the second night they have recovered from this and realise they are no longer safely cocooned in a warm, dark womb. This can mean more wakefulness, lots of feeding (normal!) and possibly crying. You might see their little eyes peeking up at you a lot in the dark. It can be quite hard as a new parent to deal with this, especially while you are recovering yourself, and you may start to worry that you are doing something wrong. Of course, we want to make sure our babies are feeding effectively, but I want you to be a little prepared for a rocky second night. It feels hard at the time, but I promise you it will get better.

If you are breastfeeding, your little one is working really hard to stimulate your milk supply. It is all about survival for them – your colostrum smells familiar; the taste is said to mimic amniotic fluid. They want to be close to your heartbeat and your voice, which is also familiar to them. It's a time of big adjustment for everyone, but I want you to know that your baby isn't broken and you aren't doing anything wrong. You might not get a lot of sleep, but as hard as it is, it is normal.

# FEEDING YOUR BABY

Ideally, your baby should go longer than two to three hours between feeds until they have regained their birth weight (this should be monitored in your baby's red book by the community midwives) and tends to be measured regularly until they sign you off two weeks after birth. If, for some reason, you have not been visited, it is imperative that you contact your community midwife team. Please don't worry about being a nuisance – it is important for you and your baby's care. Your midwife or paediatric team can give you advice on a feeding plan if your baby needs some extra help or more regular feeds.

It is important that we feed our babies really regularly during the day and night, so do keep an eye on nappy output and consider waking your baby from naps or during the night if they have not yet regained their birth weight. Do not feel bad about waking them from a nap and always check their nappy output. Consult your midwife or health visitor if you have any concerns.

Keep in mind that babies feed for other reasons than hunger, such as when they are cold, have a wet nappy or just want to be close to you.

## Breastfeeding and sleep

All small babies will wake at night to feed, but if you are establishing breastfeeding, I want you to know what is normal and what is going on with your little one's sleep. For some, breastfeeding can be a convenient and relaxing way to get your baby off to sleep. However, if you are struggling, it might be even more difficult to feel rested. You might need some help to get your breastfeeding journey started. Seeking out some skilled feeding support can really make a difference.

You might have been told that breastfed babies don't sleep well, which is both unhelpful and misleading. You can practise all the advice and techniques in this book, regardless of your feeding method.

———————————————

Breast milk is pretty magical stuff. Not only is it tailored to your baby, full of antibodies and readily available, but it also contains hormones that make baby sleepy.

In the first few months (and possibly beyond), it is very normal for your baby to fall asleep at the breast and to need the breast to get back to sleep. It is often the easiest way to settle them. This doesn't mean that you can't practise other ways if you are finding it too demanding, however, or get your partner involved in settling your baby. You can work on sleep whenever you want, optimising both your own and your baby's sleep.

You might find that during the night you want to share the burden of night wakings a little – this could mean your partner winding or settling baby after you have fed them. Or it might just mean your partner caring for you during the night, while you feed baby – getting you a glass of water, a cup of tea or slice of toast (you get the gist).

As your baby grows, you will find it easier to feed at night-time. When they are newborn, you might need to be quite 'hands-on' with their latch (they are learning just as you are), which can mean turning on the light and fully sitting up. Making sure you are comfortable and supported is important. Positioning is everything. This means you will likely be quite 'awake' for the feeds in the early days. I recommend using an amber reading light (see page 73) to save yourself from being stimulated by a bright light.

Once your baby gets a bit more efficient at the breast and they are physically larger, your night feeds will get a bit quicker and easier. This means that hopefully you can do a quick feed and head back to sleep. I remember many nights in those early days trying to keep myself awake while I fed – those newborn feeds can feel like an eternity when you desperately want to go back to sleep.

If your baby is not emptying the breast as efficiently as possible, this may mean they are not taking a full feed, which will affect their sleep. It is normal for breastfeeding to feel a little uncomfortable, but pain is not normal. It can mean that your baby isn't latching as well as they could. If you are feeling uncomfortable or in pain, make sure you seek advice with the latch and positioning of your baby as soon as possible. If your pain lasts throughout your feeds, you have misshapen nipples at the end of feeds (like a lipstick shape) or your nipple turns white, stings or is damaged, it is time to get some help.

## THE LATCH

You want baby nice and close to your body. Their nose should be in line with your nipple with their head free – don't restrict the back of their head with your hands, just cup it so it can move freely. Babies need to be able to tip their heads back – imagine drinking a can of fizzy drink! Aim to have their chin touching your breast and leading the movement. Wait until they open wide and go for it! You can try shaping your breast a bit like a burger (it really helped me to imagine a Big Mac) – they need to get a lovely big mouthful of breast tissue, not just nibbling at the edge of the patty (aka your nipple). It can be hard to remember all this during the night and let them nipple feed, but really try to get your positioning right, even if you are sleepy.

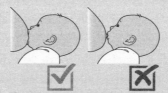

*Breastfeeding latch: good and bad*

**Breastfeeding support**

Your midwife, health visitor or local peer support group should be able to help you with breastfeeding. There may also be local drop-ins in your area – it is always worth seeing what is in your area before your baby arrives. If your baby isn't feeding as well as they could, it is going to cause more disruption to their (and your!) sleep. If you are still struggling and have the funds to do so, you can hire a lactation consultant privately. These are highly qualified breast-feeding specialists who can help with basic and complex needs. See page 283 for breastfeeding support information.

---

**BREAST COMPRESSION**

Always get a second opinion from someone qualified if you are unsure, but, in the early days, using breast compressions saved me when my babies were very small and got tired when they were feeding. This technique puts pressure on the milk ducts and can help to make feeding more efficient:

1. Support your breast with one hand – thumb on one side, fingers on the other.
2. Wait while your baby breastfeeds actively, their jaw moving all the way to their ear. When their swallowing slows, compress your breast firmly to increase milk flow and encourage swallowing. Hold it squeezed while they continue nursing actively, then release your hand.
3. Rotate your hand around the breast and repeat step 2 on different areas of the breast.

Once you feel comfortable doing so, you can try side-lying breastfeeding. I found this particularly useful after my C-sections and also when I felt especially tired. If you think you could fall asleep feeding, it is much safer to feed your baby in this position than anywhere else. You can then roll your baby onto their back and follow safe bed-sharing guidance (see page 53). If your baby has reflux (see page 88), this is also a great position as you can put them on their left side which helps work with the digestive system.

## IS YOUR BABY TONGUE-TIED?

Tongue tie can affect feeding and sleep. The way our tongue sits in the mouth when we are asleep affects our breathing. If your baby has a tongue tie it can encourage mouth breathing. If you suspect your little one may have a tongue tie, you can ask for a referral for a feeding assessment. It is a myth that tongue tie only affects breastfed babies. It can also affect bottle-fed babies. Tongue tie can mean that your little one isn't feeding effectively, so is always hungry – if they can't latch properly to the breast or bottle, they are not able to create the airtight seal with their lips that is needed. This also means they may take in lots of air, causing discomfort. You can ask your doctor for a referral or seek a tongue tie practitioner privately for a release.

### Tongue-tied baby

*I remember speaking to one mum who told me that the first 12 weeks of her little one's life were absolute hell. She had checked with so many professionals – midwives, her GP – and friends and family, but no one could work out why her baby fed so often (and woke so often!) around the clock. She had messaged me on Instagram in a moment of desperation to ask me if I had any advice. I always suggest that parents get a second opinion if their gut says something is wrong. I recommended she check again for tongue tie with a professional. She managed to find a tongue tie practitioner in her local area who diagnosed a 'hidden tongue tie', otherwise known as a posterior tongue tie. This was separated and she did 'oral exercises' to help her baby feed with the new-found freedom, and to latch effectively. Within a matter of weeks, her little one's sleep (and feeding) had transformed. Baby was sleeping for five- to six-hour chunks at night, which was utterly life-changing when they had previously seen every hour of the night.*

## Formula feeding and sleep

For many parents, breastfeeding isn't an option. Maybe you don't want to breastfeed, you can't breastfeed or you weren't supported as you should have been and breastfeeding wasn't established. All these reasons, and many more, are valid. You never need to justify your feeding journey to anyone. Some women feel a lot of grief and guilt about not breastfeeding.

Some parents are told that their baby will sleep better if they are formula-fed, but this is not the case.

---

'Filling your baby up' is not going to make them sleep
longer or mean that they don't wake regularly in
those early days.

---

It is important that your baby is comfortable for them to sleep well. So, we want feeding to be going well. This is where wind comes in.

My number one tip for making up a bottle of formula is do not shake the bottle like a cocktail – swirl it like a fine wine! If the powder isn't dissolving, you can use a sterilised spoon to stir it. When you shake the bottle, it creates air bubbles which will enter your baby's tummy and cause wind and upset. This can cause your baby to wake up soon after they have gone off to sleep or stop them from falling asleep in the first place.

Winding your baby is also key – if your baby has wind they are going to struggle to settle and sleep soundly. Some babies are windier than others, but it's always worth ruling it out. See page 117 for more on winding.

Any first infant formula is suitable for your baby for 0–12 months (you don't need follow-on formula; this is just a clever way around marketing laws). There are, of course, different formulas on the market, but, legally, they all have to meet the same nutritional guidelines. Don't be fooled by 'hungry' infant formula. This won't make your baby sleep better – it just contains more casein than whey, which takes longer to digest. There is no evidence that it helps with sleep.

No formula is superior to another in terms of its nutritional value, but you might find that your baby seems more content on one particular brand. This is totally individual.

I recommend practising paced bottle-feeding – this means allowing baby to control the pace of their feeds, which in turn means they don't take more milk than they need, which will make them uncomfortable and harder to settle. With this technique, hold baby upright, rather than lying them flat. Just being slightly reclined rather than fully flat means that milk doesn't just come pouring into their mouths. Feeding with the bottle in a horizontal position means that baby takes down milk at a slower pace, so they get the chance to recognise they are full. You can also pause and give breaks. One of the big benefits is that baby gulps down less air, meaning less chance of 'colic' (see page 118) and less sleep disturbance.

## Combination feeding

Some parents decide to combi feed from the beginning, and others gradually add in formula over time. There are many reasons you might decide to do this – either from necessity or choice. I don't believe that changing feeding method will affect your baby's sleep, so please don't give your baby formula with this hope as you may be disappointed and risk the cons below. If in doubt, seek skilled, personalised advice.

### Pros of combi feeding

- You get a break if you are the breastfeeding parent.
- You know your baby will take a bottle if you need them to.
- For some families this means that their breastfeeding journey is extended as it feels more manageable.
- You may have been told you need to supplement with formula – but continuing with any breast milk alongside it is beneficial, so your baby gets the best of both worlds in this sense.

### Cons of combi feeding

- You risk your baby getting used to the bottle (which is easier to drink from) and rejecting the breast. This is why paced bottle-feeding is really important if you are combi feeding.
- Many parents begin combi feeding and it impacts their supply and they end up in a vicious cycle, which marks the beginning of the end of breastfeeding.
- If you are not regularly emptying the breast, you can be at risk of blocked ducts and mastitis (not fun).

## DOES YOUR BABY HAVE REFLUX?

If your baby is suffering from reflux, it can be hard for them to be comfortable enough to sleep soundly. It is important to note that some regurgitation or posseting is normal. Babies have an immature gut, so it's very common for them to 'spit up'. This can include stomach acid. Some babies are sick and it doesn't bother them at all, however, others experience lots of pain and discomfort. If your baby is suffering from reflux you should speak to your doctor, but you can do some simple things to help with sleep:

- Keep your baby upright for 30 minutes after feeds before putting them to bed. Singing a lullaby or reading a story can fill this time.
- Try giving small feeds, more often.
- Keep baby's head higher than their bottom while feeding.
- If you are bottle-feeding, you can try slowing down your feeds and winding regularly.
- Speak to your doctor or health visitor about a potential course of treatment – it's always worth trying to get to the bottom of the cause.

## INTRODUCING YOUR BABY TO OTHERS

As soon as your due date comes around, you will likely have well-meaning friends and relatives asking if baby has arrived yet. The same enthusiastic people will become people who want to visit your baby. While, of course, you may be really keen to see your friends and family straight away, I highly recommend holding back for a day or two, or, if possible, a week or three! Of course, if you need the practical help (getting home from the hospital for example) then you will need them. Also, if you are a single parent, you will need a good support system in place.

My rules, for the first few weeks at least, are that anyone visiting is there to help – to cook, to clean or to feed you. It might sound harsh, but you are going to possibly be the most vulnerable you have ever been. You shouldn't need to pretend things are normal when you have just gone through a major experience with your body – you are looking after a small human being and you are sleep-deprived. The one thing that we need during these first few months of our baby's lives, therefore, is lots of support – whether that's from our partner, our families or our friends.

In many cultures around the world, it is commonplace that, during this early postpartum period, the mother is 'mothered' by those around her – an extended network of family and neighbours who provide food for the mother and help settle and care for baby so that she can rest. Your rest and recovery are the most important things in this experience. It seems that in Western culture we have forgotten the importance of rest – and we have 'lost' our villages, with many of us living far away from family and friends. In not-so-long days gone by, and in fact when my mum had me, she stayed in hospital for over a week – a whole week of someone else helping you with your baby . . . imagine! Our NHS in the UK simply doesn't have the capacity to do this anymore. I was shocked that even after my C-section with my second baby they told me that, if I really wanted to, I could go home the next day. In fact, the only reason I didn't was due to a delay in the paperwork to get us out. I was quite grateful in the end. There is no other major surgery we would undertake and be sent home the next day, other than childbirth.

Even with the most straightforward of vaginal births, you need to rest. You do not need to be entertaining, passing the baby around or putting on your make-up (unless you want to, of course, and some do). Most of us would be better off resting up in bed or on the sofa, cuddling our babies and being looked after by someone else.

I want you to truly preserve your opportunities to rest. Don't allow guests to come over and keep you awake when you could be napping. There may also be the expectation that you wake your baby so that visitors can see them. Newborns sleep a lot! It is unfair to expect you to disrupt your little one for someone else's benefit. If your baby needs to feed, they need to feed. Don't feel like you shouldn't be doing this because of prying eyes. If your baby is tired and needs to nap, settle them down. If you need to nap, try to make that happen.

### Advocating for yourself

You are likely to receive lots of advice from others in these early weeks, but it might not suit your family. Each baby and each family are so different, so it is important that we communicate our needs. But advocating for ourselves can be hard.

You can miss out on a lot of rest in the first few months as you sacrifice it for others, so embrace the cuddles and the bonding time with your baby, but it doesn't mean you need to sacrifice your well-being. Prioritising your rest and your baby's sleep can feel difficult when well-meaning friends and family suggest visits and activities which are at odds with that. Learning to advocate for yourself and your child starts here.

Don't allow anyone to make you feel like you should be acting like everything is normal when it feels like it isn't. Do see people on your terms, who help you, keep you company in the way that you want and make you feel better after seeing them. Your long-lost aunt who expects tea and sandwiches can wait. Your friend who has planned a lunch out that you don't feel ready for can wait. The friend who brings you a home-cooked meal and takes the baby for a walk while you sleep can stay.

Hold your boundaries and protect your sleep,
recovery and rest.

## SLEEP AND POSTNATAL DEPRESSION (PND)[1]

It can be quite common for new parents to struggle with their mental health after birth. If you are struggling with anxiety, PND or you just don't feel yourself, there is no shame in needing help.

The symptoms of PND and sleep deprivation can look very similar:

- tearfulness
- feeling numb
- anxiety
- irritability
- struggling to bond with baby
- withdrawing from friends and family
- intrusive thoughts
- fear of being alone
- struggling to focus
- obsessive thoughts
- lack of appetite
- feeling anxious
- low mood
- insomnia

It seems to work two ways: sometimes parents are dismissed, and well-meaning friends and relatives will tell them they 'just need a good night's sleep', when in actual fact there is more at play. Other times the commonly accepted sleep deprivation can mask PND when parents are really struggling and need help.

There are, of course, parents who do just need a good night's sleep and who would be able to cope far better with their feelings if they were sleeping better. Mental health and sleep are bidirectional – mental health issues can have a detrimental impact on our sleep, but equally lack of sleep can exacerbate mental health issues. The research does suggest that there is an association between the sleep quality of women who had given birth in the past few months and symptoms of PND.

A good night's sleep alone won't solve PND, but it may help you feel more equipped to face it and get the help that you need. PND and anxiety are conditions that you need to address with a medical professional (see page 284 for details on where you can seek help).

## EXPERT HELP

Talking of postnatal support, you may want to consider hiring help if you are in a position to do so. Such help can be particularly useful if you have no friends or family nearby and no other options for help. Before I had kids, I had no idea that these things existed or the difference between these options. I thought they were for the super-rich or lazy parents. How wrong I was! I really do feel that, if you have the means (and some of these options are not as expensive as you may think), there is absolutely no shame in getting some support, whether that's regular or sporadic. I often say save the money on all the gadgets, clothes and baby products and put it towards practical help instead. Obviously, you need to pick someone who fits well with your family and who is fully trained, but these people know how to support you and give you a break. Of course, it's also not for everyone.

### Doula

The main difference between a doula and a maternity nurse is that doulas tend to focus on the mother – they are there to help you – and maternity nurses focus more on the baby. There is naturally a lot of crossover between the two! In my experience, doulas are there to take the emotional weight off – they might get involved with household chores, other children and help establish breast-feeding. However, they all work differently so just make sure you are clear on the kind of support you are looking for.

### Maternity nurse

A maternity nurse will likely stay overnight with you and help set-tle baby, change baby and potentially look at getting you into a routine when baby is ready. If you are breastfeeding, they will bring baby to you to feed and then wind and settle baby for you. If you are bottle-feeding, they will do the feeds for you. Like all pro-fessions, some are better than others. Some people will hire a maternity nurse for a few nights, while others will use them for the entire first few months.

### Night nanny

This is someone who you tend to pay on an ad hoc basis to care for your baby overnight – this is useful if you are at the end of your tether and just want a night's sleep. If it's something that appeals to you, always get references and do your due diligence. It's okay to interview someone first and ask them about their ethos and approach.

### Sleep consultants

Of course, there are also sleep consultants like me and my team. We help with the process of sleep training your baby. This is usually offered over the age of six months as formal sleep training is not age-appropriate for younger babies. With younger babies, we are also more likely to come across allergies and health conditions that might not have been diagnosed or dealt with – this will mean referring you back elsewhere and halting our work together. You can, however, absolutely work on shaping your little one's sleep before this time, but most families find they get the most benefit when working one-to-one with a sleep consultant post-six months old. This is also the time when parents may be considering moving baby into their own room and will be thinking about starting solids and having more of a regular routine. From my years of working with individual families, I see the most dramatic results with babies who are over six months. If you find a sleep consultant who also helps with younger babies, ensure that the methods they practise are age-appropriate.

Sleep consultants are also trained to notice any red flags, anything concerning about your baby and we can give really practical advice on tailored routines and ways of settling (see Chapter 8).

## A helping hand

*One of the couples I worked with was two women, caring for their toddler and newborn baby. They had been on a long journey to have this child, and all their friends and family were very excited. The birth mum had a very long labour and an assisted delivery and had really suffered post-birth – she was struggling to get any rest as she was in so much discomfort. Her lovely partner was doing her best, but she tended to end up dealing with their toddler, who was quite sensitive and demanded a lot of attention. They had so many visitors who wanted to come and see them, but they had to keep turning them away as it felt too stressful. This left both parents feeling isolated. The birth mum told me that by day ten she had hit breaking point and hired a postnatal doula. This immediately took the pressure off their family – the doula helped with their toddler (who grew to absolutely love her!), cooked meals and supported breastfeeding. She also helped them understand the importance of rest (for the whole family). Having this extra support was a lifeline for them.*

## RELAXING WHILE YOUR BABY NAPS

Some people's instinct is to use the time that their baby is napping to catch up on chores, but this can quickly become exhausting. In the early days, if you are able, I recommend trying to take a nap at the same time as your baby at least once per day. This might be best taken in your bedroom. Don't beat yourself up if you are someone who can't nap during the day. Instead, lie down and practise some simple relaxation exercises during these moments. This doesn't have to be anything complex – simply take some time for yourself, where you lie down and take some deep breaths into your belly. Try breathing in for a count of four seconds, and out for eight seconds. You can also try holding on to that breath for a few seconds before you breathe out.

When I do this myself, I say a little mantra 'begin again' and I repeat this on each breath. It sounds corny, but our breath is what gives us life – breathing new life into our bodies is a chance to start afresh. Maybe you lost your temper with your partner, maybe you felt frustrated by your baby and now feel guilty. Whatever is going on, this moment of calm with just you and your breath is a chance to 'begin again'.

If this isn't for you, listening to a podcast, an audio-book or some music – or whatever you find relaxing – can give your mind the break that it needs and help you to relax. If you still feel like it would help you to catch up on housework during these windows, try to choose just one small chore to complete each nap to keep your energy levels from plummeting.

## YOUR RECOVERY

How well you recover – or don't recover – from the physical effects of pregnancy and birth will affect the quality of your sleep and your ability to rest. This then becomes a vicious cycle, as not getting enough rest and good-quality sleep may hinder your recovery. There are many things you can do to aid your recovery.

### Take vitamins

You should be taking vitamin D at the very least as it is crucial for our sleep, recovery and making the most of our 'window of opportunity' to sleep. Most of us are deficient in the UK, and certainly after childbirth our levels can be low – even lower in the winter months. If your vitamin D levels are low, it can have a negative impact on your sleep, among many other functions in the body, but certainly your recovery in general. If your baby is breastfed, they should also be taking a vitamin D supplement, irrespective of whether you are taking one. If your baby has more than 500ml of first infant formula per day, they don't need a supplement. It includes vitamins A, C and D among the other nutrients that your baby needs.

If your doctor or midwife has advised you to, you may also be taking iron – it is important to keep on top of this. Low iron can also cause sleep disruption – it is always worth checking this with a blood test for you or your baby if you are concerned.

### Eat a healthy diet

Having a varied, balanced diet wherever possible will also help your recovery. When we are sleep-deprived, we crave sugar and carbs. I'd lean into this – it is not the time to deprive yourself – but try to make sure you are getting some protein, good fats, vegetables and fruit in too. To support the repair of our tissues we need good protein, nutrients and to drink enough water. I highly recommend having a big bottle of water by your bed, within easy reach, that you can sip on. Easy-to-grab snacks by the bed for night feeds can be great too – think bananas, nuts or crackers for a quick energy fix.

While it is important to include healthy foods in our diets, please do not think about losing weight or 'bouncing back'. You have just had a baby. Restriction of food is never a good idea. You do not want to wake up hungry in the night because you haven't eaten enough during the day!

Listen to your body and nourish it whenever you can,
just as you nourish and feed your baby.

### Get outside

While we should rest as much as possible, we want our bodies to be strong and to function at their best. Moving a little and trying to get outside in the natural light will help your sleep. Try a short walk initially – however far you can manage without pushing it, even if it's a few minutes the first time. I shuffled down the street on day five after my third C-section and that was enough! But that feeling of the fresh air on my face was enough to blow away the cobwebs. Natural light during the day helps to regulate our internal body clocks. It's also helpful to teach your newborn the difference between day and night (see page 72).

### Have a physical health check

If we are in physical discomfort while we are in bed and there is inflammation in the body (injury), this is going to affect our quality of sleep. I highly recommend seeing a women's health physio postnatally if you are able to. You can do this as soon as you feel ready, or as soon as you can get an appointment. Your GP should be able to refer you too. If you have pelvic pain, any kind of incontinence, a diastasis (separation of your abdominals) or any other challenge in this area, then you can get a referral. If you would like to find a women's health physio privately, you can find a directory on the 'Squeezy' app, which is also a great app to help you with your pelvic floor exercises (squeezyapp.com).

---

Don't suffer through pain because you think it's 'normal'. Get help.

---

Regaining your core strength and recovering from pregnancy and childbirth can be a slow process. I myself have suffered from pelvic girdle pain for many years. I have found that strengthening the supporting muscles of the pelvis, while having manual therapy, is the best way forward (see Useful Resources, page 285).

### Get help

To recover physically, we really do need as much rest as possible, so anything you can do to help that is worth it. Do whatever is in your power to make your life easier. Meal delivery services, cooking and batch freezing in advance, or asking friends for dinners, lunches and snacks when they ask you if you need anything, can all give you more time for rest. Get a cleaner if you can, even if it's just once. A voucher for breastfeeding support, sleep support, cooking or cleaning is worth its weight in gold too. I have been to a lot of baby showers in my time, but I never see these things on the gift list. I truly believe these are the gifts you would value the most. You probably have all the babygrows that you need by now, so although they are a really lovely gift, I would ask for these practical things I have mentioned instead.

### Have a birth debrief

If you had a traumatic birth, I highly recommend getting a birth debrief. Dealing with any kind of trauma can have an impact on your sleep. It is hard to relax and switch off if you are processing something very stressful. You may even be afraid to sleep, in case you dream about your experience. A birth debrief is an opportunity to speak to a doctor or midwife about your birth, run through what happened and ask any questions you have. There are also private practitioners who offer this service. Your GP can also refer you, or you can self-refer via IAPT, if you need to speak to a trained therapist.

### GETTING BACK TO SLEEP AFTER NIGHT FEEDS

If you struggle to get back to sleep after night feeds, I highly recommend practising some deep breathing, listening to an audiobook or getting out of bed to do some gentle stretches. If you are tossing and turning for a long time, you might want to change your location, even for a moment. This can help your brain to reset. Getting out of bed and making a snack or a warm drink can help.

You don't need to be a yoga expert to do breathing exercises. Your breath belongs to you, and you can do this however you want. When we slow down our breathing, we send a message to our nervous system to calm down, so it can just be a case of consciously slowing your breathing. You can do this by breathing out for a longer time than when you breathe in – for example, breathe in for four, hold it for a moment, then breathe out for eight.

You may be in the habit of scrolling through your phone to look at social media or shop online while feeding during the day, but try not to do this during the night as this will stimulate your brain and tell you it's time to wake up (see page 31). You may also end up making purchases you don't really need! I once bought something on Amazon during a night feed that I totally forgot about until it turned up the next day!

Some people find watching TV really comforting at night, especially if you are feeling lonely. If you find that you struggle to get back off to sleep, it's best to keep the TV and other screens off. Keeping things calm and dark is best for sleep.

## WHEN A BABY SLEEPS FOR LONGER PERIODS

You might be one of the lucky ones whose baby is sleeping for long periods. By this I mean longer than a few hours in a row. It is normal for newborns to wake very often, but it can also be normal for them to sleep for a number of hours in a row (this is less common, and comes down to luck of the draw). Both can cause worry for many parents, especially in these early days.

I want you to know that as long as your baby is happy, has periods of time when they are alert and they are gaining weight then I wouldn't be concerned (if they are waking after very short periods and seem very uncomfortable, I would consult your GP or health visitor). It's always good to be mindful of baby's nappy output and their weight. If your baby is back to their birth weight (your community midwife should be monitoring this in your baby's red book if you are in the UK), then you no longer need to wake your baby for night feeds. I would, however, consider waking baby if they have slept for too long (that is, more than two to three hours) during the day. You really don't want your baby to sleep through daytime feeds. I am often asked how to wake a baby – I would gently pick them up and see if they rouse. If they are particularly sleepy you may need to undress them and change their nappy to get them to wake up.

There are some reasons why your baby may still be quite sleepy – jaundice can cause this, as can an infection. Also, if babies are too hot it can make them sleepy – this is also a SIDS risk (see page 64) so make sure your baby is dressed appropriately for the temperature during the day and at night. If you are ever concerned about your baby, always speak to your midwife, health visitor or GP. If your baby is unresponsive, then you need urgent care by phoning 999 (in the UK).

I hope this chapter has given you a sense of what to expect in this 'fourth trimester' and how you can help yourself to get more rest. Let's now look at ways you can get to know and understand your baby's sleep needs and begin some sort of 'routine' if you want to.

# 6

# FINDING YOUR RHYTHM

As you spend the days, weeks and months getting to know your baby, you will get to know their sleepy cues. Each baby is different, but you may see them frown, avert their gaze, become fussy, yawn, cry . . . want to feed . . . There are so many, but your baby will have their own individual set of cues. Don't worry if you feel like you don't know them yet, you will do soon!

If you are unsure or can't seem to distinguish any clear signs, just have a think about how long they have been happily awake for and see if you can see a pattern emerging to your days. Do bear in mind that some of these signals are interchangeable – babies can fuss and cry when they are tired, hungry or even just bored. It used to drive me wild when strangers or friends and family made comments about my babies like, 'She looks tired', when in actual fact she had just woken from a long nap! Remember – you know your baby best. It is always a bit of trial and error, which is why having a rhythm to your day helps – this makes it a little easier to read your baby as you have a rough idea of when they might be tired or hungry.

## ANCHOR YOUR DAY

With a first baby, families often end up starting the day at different times. This might work for you, but it can feel chaotic. If you only do one simple thing regarding 'routine', you can simply aim to begin and end your day at roughly the same time. (It can feel quite painful to set an alarm, but you don't need to be completely rigid about it.) If you already have children, this is somewhat a moot point as you will probably already be up and about for nursery or the school run – the luxury of late starts may already be a distant memory.

I generally find babies and children are naturally early risers, compared to many adults, so a wake-up time of anything between 6 and 7.30am works well. A bedtime between approximately 6.30 and 8.30pm works well for most little ones too. That way you have roughly a 12-hour day to fit in naps and feeds. Don't get too worried about when these happen if it feels stressful, but the simple act of beginning your day at the same time each day will mean that, in theory, you should see a natural pattern begin to appear.

Bear in mind that sleep should be supervised in the evenings until six months according to safer sleep guidance (see Chapter 4). 'Bedtime' doesn't necessarily mean your baby is separated from you. You can settle them down in their Moses basket in the front room with you if you like or their crib in your bedroom if you are going to be with them. This is a chance for an early night, to read a book, listen to a podcast or watch TV. I do find that if you are already 'ready' for bed early yourself, you will find it much easier to have an early night. An early bedtime can be so beneficial for you if you are still experiencing night waking.

---

Get into your pyjamas early on, feed and settle baby, and then you can enjoy some peace and quiet.

---

If your little one is still cluster feeding (wanting more frequent, shorter feeds over a few hours, usually in the evening), getting ready for bed early can be transformative – sometimes the act of you relaxing and being ready for rest yourself gives your baby an opportunity to wind down and be ready for bed too. Some of us are natural night owls, so it can feel really hard to go to bed early and sacrifice our much-needed time to ourselves, but remember, this is a short period in your life, and it will get better. In the coming months, you will get your evenings back.

As your little one's circadian rhythm (see page 29) begins to appear towards the end of the 'fourth trimester', anchoring your day will become even more important.[1] Their internal clocks, along with sleep pressure (see page 29), will align and means that beginning a regular nap routine becomes easier, and more important. This doesn't mean you need to stress about naps, but if you can find a good balance of daytime sleep, it will really help your baby to be well-rested, happy and to thrive.

## YOUR BABY'S PATTERNS

You might find that anchoring your day is enough for you right now, but there is more we can do! As your baby grows in these coming weeks you might notice a pattern emerging. Their first nap of the day might just become a bit more predictable. If, for example, your day starts at 7am, your baby might be ready for their first nap at around 8/8.15am (this is just an example – this could be different depending on your baby's sleep needs). If you keep that same wake-up time (roughly), then you will start to be able to plan your day a little. Perhaps you could go for a walk at the same time each day or have baby sleep in their Moses basket while you have breakfast.

So many parents worry that a routine will be restrictive, when in fact I believe it opens you up to be able to plan your day. You know when baby is going to be awake and happy to receive visitors. You know when it is a good time to take them out to a baby class – tired or hungry babies aren't going to be receptive to baby rhyme time! It also becomes *your* routine, as much as theirs. I am a big fan of following your baby but also allowing time for yourself during the day and to get a breather. Even if you practise 'contact naps' (when your baby naps on you) or naps on the go, you can still plan your day around these. Depending on the weather, you might find that you really enjoy having a regular daily walk outside with your baby.

Having said all this, if you don't see a pattern emerging just yet, don't worry. See page 142 for how to start working on a solid routine with your baby.

## SLEEP NEEDS

Parents often want to know how much their baby *should* be sleeping at certain stages. The table below is a guide, but there really is no absolute gold standard when it comes to sleep totals. There will always be babies who need much more, or much less, sleep than this, so, as with anything, take it with a pinch of salt (in fact, we should note that sleep totals do seem to vary quite a bit country to country too, which is fascinating).

| Age | Average hours of sleep in 24 hours | Average number of naps in 24 hours |
|---|---|---|
| 0–3 months | 14–17 | 4–5 |
| 4–6 months | 13–16 | 3–4 |
| 6–9 months | 12–15 | 2–3 |
| 10–18 months | 11–14 | 1–2 |

## BEGINNING A BEDTIME ROUTINE

You can think about introducing a regular, predictable bedtime routine as soon as you like. This isn't set in stone, and the time of day may vary slightly, but it's a way of preparing your baby for sleep time. Babies learn repetition very quickly and find comfort in knowing what is coming next.

Babies tend to be nocturnal when they are first born, but, after some weeks, it can benefit the whole family to try to get them to bed a little earlier than you. There is no hard and fast rule about exactly at what age to do this (and I believe it is different culturally for each family), but *most* babies benefit from going to bed before 8pm by around three months of age. Of course, we need to practise safe sleep practices, which means sharing our sleep space with our babies for at least the first six months. Many parents ask me how they should approach this. Here is my advice:

1. You can implement a gentle bedtime routine as soon as you feel ready. This simply means doing a series of things in the same order at a similar time each evening. For example, this could be a bath, a massage, milk, a cuddle and down to bed. Babies love repetition and predictability.

2. When I say 'down to bed' you have a few options. You could put baby 'down to bed' in their Moses basket in your front room while you watch TV (and transfer them to your bedroom later). You could put baby 'down to bed' in their Moses basket or crib in your bedroom and you go to bed with them (for high sleep needs parents or those with early risers, this works well).

3. You might go to bed with them, but stay up – watching an iPad or reading a book for example (this is where a sleep-friendly coloured light can be really useful, I prefer amber – see page 73).

4. You might take turns with your partner to go to bed with baby.

5. If you want a break, you could enlist a babysitter, friend or family member to sit with baby.

6. While we want to protect our babies by following this rule, please don't think that it means you can't pop to the loo or get a snack or something else that you need. Guidance is important but there must be some flex, especially if you are on your own.

*Of course*, as I always say, if going to bed later with your baby works for you and your family, you don't need to change it. Newborns, especially, tend to be a bit more flexible with bedtimes. It also depends on the temperament of your baby, which you will get to know as they grow. I find that babies tend to get particularly over-tired and fractious from around three months onwards if they stay up late with their parents.

## BATHING YOUR BABY

Making a bath part of your baby's bedtime routine can help for when they begin to get fussy in the evenings. The warm water is relaxing and distracts them from any discomfort they might be experiencing. It is also lovely for them to have your undivided attention as you talk to them and wash their skin. You can even take a bath with your baby – just be mindful not to have the water too hot and to avoid carrying your baby while you're stepping into or out of the bath. Co-bathing is great for unsettled babies who won't seem to calm.

If you don't want to bath your baby every night then I still advise taking them into the bathroom and doing a top and tail wash with warm water and cotton wool or a wash-cloth, so that they still experience this as one of the predictable steps of their routine. The other steps could be a lullaby, a massage, cuddles, a feed and then into their Moses basket or crib. Putting your baby into their sleeping bag or swaddle is also a step. Don't underestimate the power of repetition and familiarity. (But make sure you stop swaddling by 16 weeks at the latest – see page 124 – or as soon as your baby shows signs of rolling.)

### Your baby's individual needs

Having a bedtime routine that aligns with your baby being sleepy enough is also important. Making sure that you aren't trying to put them down before they are ready can make your life much easier. Although I have mentioned earlier on about babies benefiting from an 'early' bedtime, this could vary quite a bit from baby to baby. I find that anything from 6.30 to 8.30pm works for this age group.

---

You need to make sure you leave enough time from the end of their last nap to when you are putting them down for bedtime, otherwise you will have an unnecessary battle on your hands.

---

How long your baby is happily awake will vary from baby to baby, but most need to be awake from 5/5.30pm for a 7pm bedtime for example, but play around with it – your baby might need less or more time. If you are trying to bring bedtime earlier, you will definitely need to reduce that last nap or make it earlier.

If your baby is going to bed even later with you, and that works for you and your family, it is absolutely fine to continue to do that for now. You will find, as they get bigger, more alert and more active, they will naturally go down to bed a little earlier.

## PRACTISING SETTLING TO SLEEP

It is normal for your baby to need your help to get to sleep. It is also normal if your baby does this on their own – there really is no right or wrong. If you are happy with how your days and nights are going and how you settle your baby, you do not need to change anything. There is no rush to do this, or a rush for independence. It might seem that baby sleep is a race, but it really isn't. We can go at our baby's pace. However, you may find that, when you have a more predictable day and are getting to know your baby, you might want to see if they can settle themselves. In these early months I see this a little like an experiment – unless you give it a shot, you won't know the outcome. If the recipe isn't quite right, you can change it. And you can always return and try later.

Watch your baby's tiredness cues and take them to their sleep space to settle them down. You may be doing this at bedtime (which, in fact, I recommend as you have sleep pressure – see page 29 – on your side!) or at naptime. Aim to put your baby into their sleep space either awake or a little sleepy. As they grow, we will be aiming to put them down fully awake so that they are aware of their environment. There is nothing wrong with putting your baby down fully asleep, especially if they are one of the ones who sleep well regardless, but, in my practice, I have noticed that babies who are able to get themselves to sleep at the beginning of their sleep time are more likely to be able to connect their sleep cycles without assistance during naps and during the night. It is very normal for smaller babies not to do this – it is a skill that often comes much later.

If your baby fusses briefly when you put them down, it is okay to take a step back and observe what they do. If they begin to cry, pick them up, comfort them and try again, or you can abandon your practice session for this time. You have not failed; you have simply given it a go. You can return to your usual way of helping baby to sleep. There is more time to help baby fall asleep on their own at a later stage. You can keep trying occasionally across the next few weeks or try once a day. Or you might wait until baby is six months – I will give you more guidance on this later.

---

Babies who are able to get themselves to sleep at the beginning of their sleep time are more likely to be able to connect their sleep cycles without assistance during naps.

---

### Sleep cues

You will grow to learn your own baby's sleep cues over time as you get to know each other. Some babies give really clear signals, while others can be a little more subtle. You'll start to pick up on what is unique to your baby, but these are general signals that babies give:

| Early signs | 'I'm ready now' | 'I'm really ready now – please help!' |
|---|---|---|
| Staring into the distance, turning into your body or looking away from stimulating situations | Yawning – an obvious one as we recognise this in ourselves. For some babies, a yawn is one of the last sleepy signals they give, while for others it happens a bit earlier | Jerky arm/leg movements or seeming restless |
| Pink eyebrows/ furrowed brow | Wanting to feed – this needs to be taken in context. Your baby may just be due a feed, but some babies seek the comfort of sucking to fall asleep and will ask you for a feed | Crying |
| Grouchy | Rubbing eyes or ears | Sucking on fingers |
| Unsettled | Grizzly | Frowning or furrowed brow |
| | Difficulty focusing | Becoming rigid |
| | Fluttering eyelids | Hands in fists |

## THE IMPORTANCE OF THE PAUSE

It is important to note that babies sometimes make a lot of noise in their sleep. This happens when they are in active sleep, and often between their sleep cycles. Of course, we need to be responsive to our babies, but sometimes we can be on 'high alert' and respond too quickly, thinking that baby is awake, when in fact they are still asleep. This can result in us waking our babies when they would have carried on sleeping otherwise. Your baby may moan, groan, pass wind, wriggle and make little noises, but it doesn't necessarily mean that they need you in that moment.

Becoming a parent comes with a huge weight of responsibility, and naturally we are on 'high alert' when our babies are first born – this is an important protective instinct and designed so that we feed our babies and keep them safe. However, often this 'high alert' continues into the following months and means we can find it hard to switch off from these little noises and come to the realisation that our babies don't always need us in these moments.

---

Pausing for a moment before you reach into that crib or cot can be beneficial. It is always worth waiting, reflecting and seeing what happens.

---

Your baby may just surprise you; you have nothing to lose.

When I had my first baby, I literally jumped out of bed even if she flinched. Looking back, I felt very anxious that I needed to be doing the very best job I could do, and that meant I had to be on the ball. I didn't realise that, by doing this, I was actually doing the opposite of what we wanted to achieve. I was overbearing when settling her and I was disturbing her sleep. Noises, movement and even our babies being vocal can be a really normal part of active sleep. If we step in too soon, we can wake them up fully or stop them going into their next sleep cycle. It was also very stressful for both me and my husband. It meant that, even with the sleep I was getting, it felt like I was sleeping with half an ear and half an eye open.

## WAKE WINDOWS

A 'wake window' is how long your little one has been comfortably awake for before they need to go to sleep – either for a nap or bedtime. There is no official guidance on them, which is why you will often find differing lengths in the guides that you find online. They are simply what consultants like me have noticed during their practice.

Wake windows can be really helpful, but don't get too hung up on them. Each baby is different – some need much less sleep than others, some need much more, and some are somewhere around the middle. It is about observing your baby and seeing what works and keeping up with their growth and development. As they grow, they will be able to stay awake longer – it's important to keep on top of this otherwise we risk trying to get our babies to nap, or go to bed, before they are ready. Personally, I stopped worrying about wake windows at around eight weeks onwards for my second and third babies – this is when they fell into more of a rhythm to their days anyway.

Some people find wake windows confusing and stressful. If this is you, feel free to ditch them and not worry about it! If you want a rough steer, then the awake times below are a good guide, but please don't worry if your baby's sleep doesn't match these:

- **0–1 month:** 45 minutes, but can be less
- **1–2 months:** 45–60 minutes
- **2–3 months:** 1–1.5 hours

I find wake windows to be far more useful in the early weeks and months than later on. Certainly, once your baby is six months and you are introducing solids, a more predictable routine seems to work best for most babies.

## PLAYTIME AND TUMMY TIME

Adding in some physical movement and some stimulating play to your day can benefit both you and your baby and improve your sleep.

As the weeks pass by, you will notice that your baby is becoming more alert and able to stay awake for longer during the day. They might also start getting bored. This is something that can happen quite quickly and take us by surprise. Our babies suddenly need entertaining. It is quite common for parents to think that their little ones are tired, when in fact they need a change of scene or some other play or stimulation. I am not talking about a full-on amateur dramatics show or complicated things. It can be as simple as singing songs, physical play and getting out of the home regularly.

I am a big fan of getting out and about twice a day if possible: once in the morning and once in the afternoon. If your routine doesn't allow this, then it is probably too restrictive. You also don't need to spend a lot of money on toys. Anything that is shiny, makes a noise or your baby can chew and is safe, works!

---

If your baby doesn't get mental and physical stimulation, they will not be as tired for sleep.

---

Sleep pressure will rise as the day goes on, but I find that fresh air each day and playtime really boosts this and helps them to be tired for their naps and bedtime. If you have some outside space, it is lovely to play outside if it is warm enough, or head to your local park with a blanket and some toys.

When I talk about physical play, you might wonder what on earth I mean for babies within the first few months when they can't move. One of the best things you can start with is tummy time. This is *so* beneficial for many reasons – it is a form of self-massage for your baby, working on any wind they are holding. It also helps them work on their core and upper body and neck strength. This is a precursor to rolling and crawling. Just as adults need movement in their day, our babies do too. Leaving them in 'containers' for too long during the day can slow down these developmental milestones and mean your baby is less ready for sleep. By a 'container' I mean a car seat, bouncer or buggy, where the baby is kept in an upright position and can't stretch out or practise movement.

This is not the same as a pram where your baby is in a flat position and can move easily.

### *More playtime please!*

*One of my friends asked me for a coffee to have a chat about her ten-week-old. She told me that baby Bonnie had gone from taking three to four naps, which were predictable and fairly long, to suddenly battling them and waking more at night. We had a look at her overall day and found that Bonnie was ready to be awake longer than her mum thought. She also needed a bit more stimulation. She was following the same pattern for naps as she was when she was six weeks old. As a result, Bonnie wasn't ready for sleep, so mum was rocking her or walking her for half of the day to try to get her to sleep. Then she would sleep later and longer than she needed, causing fragmented nights.*

*Instead of getting her down so soon for naps, I told Bonnie's mum to focus on introducing a bit of play – some fun noisy toys, some music and getting out for fresh air each morning and each afternoon. I advised her to relax a bit about Bonnie getting 'overtired' and lean into it. If she was awake a while longer, what was the harm? As a result, she managed to get her down to three naps, with one long one in the middle of the day. This, in turn, improved their nights. Bonnie went from waking five times per night, to only two times (once at around 11pm and once at around 3–4am, when she fed and went back off to sleep until 7am).*

If your baby doesn't like tummy time initially, take some time to build up to it. Try after a nappy change, even if it's for just 30 seconds, and you can gradually build up to longer. You can also try lying your baby on your chest or over your legs instead, lying them on their side on their playmat, or using a rolled-up towel or manufactured tummy time pillow, which are widely available for purchase.

## BABY MASSAGE

I used to teach baby massage before I trained as a sleep consultant. It is great for calming the nervous system and easing your baby's immature digestive system, and it was a favourite of mine to help with colic (see page 118). It can give you a sense of control in what can feel like an out-of-control situation.

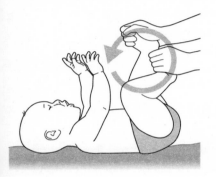

*Pedal your baby's legs in the air as if they are riding a bike.*

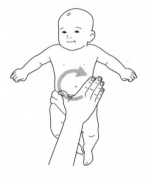

*Gently move your hands clockwise in a circular motion around baby's tummy. Be careful over the bladder.*

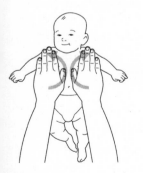

*Place your hands on your baby's chest and circle out and upwards across the shoulders.*

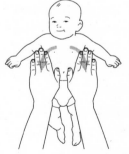

*Place your hands on baby's chest and circle outwards and in a downward motion.*

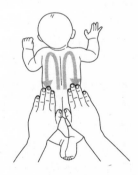

*Start at the base of your baby's spine and work upwards either side of the spine, across the shoulders, then back down the outer sides of the back.*

Massage is a lovely thing to include as part of your day at any time; it doesn't have to be bedtime. Choose a time when your baby is content and not hungry and tired. All you need is a towel, a warm room and some baby-friendly massage oil.

> I am a big fan of baby swimming and always find that my babies have been shattered and slept soundly after swimming. There may be baby swimming lessons available in your local area, or you can just take your baby with you to a local pool and create your own fun.

## STAY CURIOUS ABOUT YOUR BABY

As you begin to know your baby really well, you will have certain expectations of their naps and night-time sleeps. When they don't settle in the way you've been used to, it is time to do some detective work as there will usually be a good reason for any disruption. Try to stay open-minded and curious about your baby's sleep and their general behaviour. Sometimes they can be so baffling, and each situation requires a bit of observational work.

What is their behaviour trying to tell you?

- Are they uncomfortable?
- Are they overstimulated?
- Are there too many people around?
- Do they need to feed?
- Do they have a tummy ache?
- Is there something else underlying that I need to check out with the doctor?

While these questions are all important, we don't want to get too bogged down with anxiety and over-pathologise. So much of this can be normal baby behaviour – it is normal and common for your little one to have disturbed nights and struggle to take long naps during the day (some babies feel refreshed from a 15–30-minute nap). It doesn't necessarily mean that anything is wrong.

Trusting your gut and seeking advice when your instinct tells you something is up very valuable.

It's common for young babies, in particular, to have digestive discomfort – I am talking a mild discomfort here – and this will affect their sleep. If you feel like what your baby is experiencing isn't mild, always consult your GP or health visitor for advice.

### Does your baby need winding?

There is one thing that always seems to crop up when we least want it and becomes a real barrier to sleep – wind. It is a normal function in our body, but, for our babies, excessive wind can become a problem. If they are formula-fed, do not shake their bottle. Instead, stir it with a sterilised spoon as shaking it causes air bubbles. Make sure you are using the appropriately sized teat, and that the teat isn't full of air. You can try winding your baby halfway through or after a feed.

It is not true that breastfed babies don't need winding. It's true that *some* don't, but lots do! In theory, your baby should let you know that they are uncomfortable, but I find it is always useful to give winding a go and see what happens. We don't want to disturb a baby who is happily feeding at the breast, but for those who are fussy and crying, it's well worth it. Some babies will wake soon after being put down if they have wind. My son was one of these and he was exclusively breastfed at the time! It is always worth double-checking baby's latch if they are particularly windy.

You can try gently rubbing your baby's back, but my favourite position is to tilt your baby slightly to their left – this works with the shape of their stomachs – as wind can quite literally be trapped due to the shape of the stomach, and this is often enough to release it.

### Is your baby colicky?

'Colicky' is a phrase that describes a baby who cries a lot without an obvious cause. In my opinion, there is a cause – it is just that we don't know what it is. Of course, some crying is normal, but if you have a colicky baby you will know what we mean by 'a lot'. I believe that the common causes of colic are:

- poor latch
- tongue tie
- muscular tension from birth or delivery (here I recommend seeing a baby osteopath or chiropractor)
- allergies
- reflux (often caused by these previous things)
- wind

It is a case of doing some investigative work on behalf of your baby. Movement, getting outside, a change of scene, baby massage or co-bathing could all help to soothe a colicky baby. Ultimately, though, trying to get to the root cause is most helpful.

Colic can be brutal, but there will be an end in sight and it won't be like this forever. Always seek support and medical advice if you are concerned. There is also a charity called Cry-sis, which can be a great help during these times (see page 283).

### Has your baby been immunised recently?

In my experience, after an immunisation, your baby's sleep can be affected in a few ways. First, it is common for your baby to be a little sleepier than usual in the first 48 hours after a vaccine. This is their immune system working hard creating antibodies. Alternatively, they can wake up more than usual if they have discomfort at the site of the injection. Your baby may develop a fever after the MenB vaccine, so be sure to give them some paracetamol. In some babies you don't even notice a difference in their sleep, so you might be surprised, but be prepared to comfort your baby as usual and know that any disturbance should pass quickly. If you are ever concerned, speak to your doctor or practice nurse who can give you more information.

### Is your baby constipated?

If your baby is constipated, the stool is often hard and your baby will strain to pass it. It will cause discomfort and therefore they might struggle to sleep soundly. It is worth noting that not all babies poo every day, although this is more common after the age of six weeks, so it's not necessarily how often they go that we are concerned with, but how hard it is for them. If you are concerned that your baby may be constipated, please consult your GP or health visitor.

Baby massage (see page 115) is a great way to help get your little one's digestive system moving. Gently massage your baby's tummy in a circular motion, in a clockwise direction. You can also try 'bicycle legs', where you gently move their legs as if they are riding a bike. If your baby is formula feeding, you can give a little cooled boiled water between feeds, or if you are breastfeeding make sure that baby is feeding often enough and effectively. If in doubt, get help.

### CRYING TO COMMUNICATE

I think it is important to note that some level of crying is normal in our babies. It can feel hard and uncomfortable, but sometimes babies just suddenly find their voice (often around week three) and they are clearer with their commu-nication. Nobody likes crying, but it is an important method of communication for your baby (see page 39). If you have tried the usual things – for example, feeding and winding or a cuddle – it might just be that your baby is telling you they are tired. Be mindful of how long they have been awake and think about trying to settle them before they become overstimulated and distressed.

## WAYS TO SETTLE YOUR BABY

All these things are beneficial for you and your baby, so there is no harm in trying them:

- Hold your baby in different positions – 'tiger in the tree' and some swaying for example.

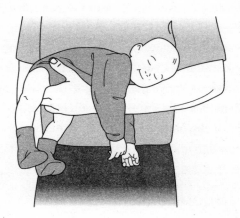

*'Tiger in the tree' hold*

- Bath your baby.
- Take your baby for a walk using a sling.
- Massage your baby (see page 115).
- If all else fails, strip both of you off and try some skin-to-skin contact (see page 78).

## Dummies, pacifiers or soothers

Whatever you call them, dummies can be a useful tool to help settle and soothe your baby. It's absolutely your choice as to whether you try one (although there are some babies who just won't take one!) – they are certainly not an essential item – and, of course, one day you will need to wean your baby off it (see page 161), but it is something you can have in your toolbox.

There are some cases where using a dummy can be especially helpful or might have even been recommended to you by a healthcare professional. For premature babies, an orthodontic dummy can help them learn to suck. For babies who suffer from reflux, a dummy can also help soothe the discomfort that they are experiencing. However, if you don't want to use a dummy then you can of course settle your reflux baby in other ways (such as rocking, walking, cuddling and so on). Sucking is very soothing for babies – whether that is on a dummy, your breast or a bottle.

The general advice for dummy use is to wait until feeding is established before introducing one. This would tend to be between four and six weeks of age. I believe you can trust your own judgement on this, but I wouldn't introduce one into the mix if you are engorged, have mastitis or are generally struggling with breastfeeding. It would be better to seek out skilled feeding support and work on your little one emptying the breast as efficiently as possible.

### HOW TO USE A DUMMY

- Offer it consistently at the beginning of sleep, both day and night (if it falls out, you don't need to replace it).
- Never use dummy cords or clips – they are a choking or strangulation risk.

- Do not force your baby to take a dummy or put anything sweet on it (yes, I have seen this in my practice!).
- Keep it clean with regular sterilising.
- Check regularly for any cracks, holes or splits as these can harbour bacteria that could make your baby sick.

You may have heard the advice that using a dummy reduces the chance of SIDS. However, this isn't cut and dry. Due to the lack of solid research around dummies, in the UK we do not recognise dummy use as a preventative measure against SIDS. What we do know is that if you are to use a dummy, it should be used for all sleep times – all naps and overnight. There are far better protective measures against SIDS (placing baby to sleep on their backs and room-sharing for six months, for example – see page 51).

There is some evidence to suggest that dummy use may increase the risk of middle ear infections, which is something to consider if your little one suffers with these (the evidence to support this is, however, limited).[2]

I always say that if dummies are helping you then great, but if they start getting in the way of a good night's sleep it is probably time to think about getting rid of them. The other option is to ride it out and wait for your little one to be old enough to put it back in themselves. The way to do this is to help them guide it back to their mouths so they learn how to put it back in, and try leaving extra dummies in their cot, so they are more likely to be able to find one.

### Thumb and finger sucking

I think thumb/finger sucking has a bad reputation and, like anything, it has its pros and cons. It is a natural way for little ones to soothe themselves, and they don't lose it like a dummy – this means that even for small babies they can find it easier to settle themselves than those who rely on a dummy (who might struggle to put it in themselves). It is often something that starts in the womb or it can start later.

I find that at around 10–12 weeks babies tend to 'find' their hands, or their thumbs specifically (if they haven't already). Therefore, I believe it is important for us to leave baby's hands uncovered when they are sleeping, particularly from around this age (if you are swaddling you are going to be thinking about removing the swaddle soon anyway – more on this below). I like to give babies the freedom to explore their hands and use them to comfort themselves. If they are stuck in mittens and swaddles this is difficult for a baby who is naturally predisposed to doing this.

Some parents are concerned about thumb and finger sucking and the impact it will have on their baby's future. Many children will naturally begin to suck their thumb less as they grow, with many giving up by the time they go to school, while others might need some encouragement. If they continue to suck their thumb or finger when their permanent teeth begin to appear, it can affect the roof of the mouth and positioning of the teeth (a dummy can also do this). In extreme cases, it can also affect the jaw and speech (a dummy can also do this too!). However, don't panic, as all these things are very dependent on how often they suck their thumb/finger, how long for and the position in the mouth. There are lots of varying factors. Some people continue to suck their thumb for years (and some well into adulthood!) and have teeth that are entirely unaffected. Others (like myself), end up wearing braces as a teenager.

For the purposes of the stage you are at right now, I really don't want you to worry about your baby sucking their thumb or using a dummy. Both are effective and easy ways for them to comfort themselves. There is no need to try to deter them from sucking their thumbs or fingers (or hands!). (And I really don't think this is possible, or kind, which is more to the point.) For the first few years of their life, it makes things far easier to just allow them to use their natural self-comforting thumb or finger than to try to fight it.

## DITCHING THE SWADDLE

Swaddling (see page 56) can be a great tool for helping your newborn sleep, making them feel more secure outside the womb and stopping their arms flailing around with their Moro (startle) reflex. However, you do need to think about stopping it by 16 weeks at the latest, or earlier than this if they are showing signs of rolling. We need to keep a close eye on our babies as some little ones start moving much sooner than others.

Part of the reason we need to ditch the swaddle is for safety – once your little one is showing signs that they are starting to roll and become mobile, it is no longer safe. However, it isn't just about sleep safety. It is also about your little one's physical development and how they settle themselves. When your baby is in their sleep space it is normal that they will start practising their new-found skills – rolling, crawling and eventually standing! If we confine them in a swaddle, they can't do these things. In theory, this could impact their motor skills.

Also, I've always thought, I like the freedom to move in bed and to find a comfortable position, and your little one is no different. You should always place them on their backs to sleep, but once they can roll both ways you can leave them to find a comfortable sleeping position. Imagine wanting to roll over in bed and something was stopping you! Babies also often soothe themselves with their hands, fingers or thumbs, as I mentioned above, and we are stopping this lovely soothing skill by using a swaddle beyond the appropriate stage.

## HOW TO GRADUALLY DITCH THE SWADDLE

- Night one: unswaddle your baby's legs.
- Night two: unswaddle one arm.
- Night three: unswaddle the other arm.
- Night four: ditch the swaddle in exchange for a sleeping bag (see page 56).

It is normal for your little one to need more support going to sleep while they are getting used to their new-found freedom. Try not to worry and allow them the space to settle.

So, you have survived the first few months and are going headlong into another period of rapid change. You will have got to know your little one's personality, sleep cues and possibly seen them develop a natural rhythm to their days. Hopefully you are feeling like you have found your feet a little more as a parent. You might have implemented a simple bedtime routine, or you might not be there just yet. You are now heading out of the fourth trimester and straight into a key period in your baby's life, where a window of sleep opportunity will open up. If you thought you'd never sleep again, you were wrong. Some solid sleep is just on the horizon. Let's go get it.

## KEY TAKEAWAYS

1. Cover the basics and decide where your baby will sleep, what they will wear and all the important safety aspects of sleep.
2. Prepare for the fourth trimester – knowing what is normal can be a great help.
3. Look after your own well-being as well as your baby.
4. Start to find a rhythm to your day – get to know your baby's cues and their wake windows.
5. Always remain curious and prepared for your baby's changing needs.

# PART 3

# 7

# THE FOUR-TO-SIX-MONTH 'PROGRESSION'

Your baby's sleep might be quite predictable now or it might have just hit the skids. Either way, you are approaching a window of golden opportunity in your baby's sleep timeline, with their sleep patterns changing dramatically – their sleep architecture is becoming more like ours as adults. This is when you might find that previous techniques you used to help your little one to get to sleep may no longer be serving you. Your peaceful sleeper may now be waking each hour, taking short naps and struggling to settle at any time of the day. Or maybe the way that you settled them previously isn't working anymore.

---

Rocking to sleep, feeding to sleep or whatever you do to help your baby off to the land of nod isn't a problem, until it becomes a problem for you.

---

If it feels unsustainable, unpleasant or frustrating and you want to change it, this is the time. This chapter is all about supporting you with that change and making the most of this golden opportunity to get a better night's sleep. From four months onwards we can start to gently shape our little one's sleep and, if you want to, you can start 'sleep training' at six months old. I am going to go on to define what that means, what our options are and how to choose the right path for you and your baby later. It is important to me that you have all the information so that you can make an informed choice about how you tackle any sleep struggles you may be experiencing, and to do so with confidence.

## THE 'FOUR-MONTH SLEEP REGRESSION'

You may have heard of this mystical milestone in your baby's sleep timeline or you may not have, but it is much talked about in the sleep world, and possibly by parents you know. I want to reassure you that it isn't a 'regression' at all. It's a progression in your baby's development. It's the only time that their sleep changes in a biological sense. Also, the change is permanent (in a biological sense), but that permanence doesn't mean that your baby won't ever sleep again. I don't really like the word regression because it sounds like your baby is going backwards, when the absolute opposite is happening. It isn't, however, something that we need to live in fear of. It is a natural, biological process and your baby's brain will do all the work.

With this change, the newborn sleep/wake cycle is replaced with more complex phases of sleep, more like that of an adult. Both babies and adults either wake or briefly stir between these sleep cycles (even if we don't remember or are not aware of it). This is where your baby's new-found increased awareness of their environment often comes into play!

This stage is called the 'four-month regression' because it tends to happen around that time, but it could happen earlier, or even later – the ballpark age for this change to occur is between three and five months old. You might, in fact, not even notice a change. Some parents are dreading this and looking for signs of it the day their little one turns four months, but nothing perceptible happens.

Don't worry about it if you haven't noticed a change – there is nothing you should be doing to 'make' it happen. If you have been busy setting the solid foundations for sleep that I have spoken about earlier, or if you have a baby who has a relaxed temperament, you might not need to do anything at all, or even have to consider it.

> **HAS YOUR BABY'S SLEEP CHANGED?**
>
> - You might notice that your baby suddenly finds it hard to switch off and seems to 'fight' sleep.
> - You might find that things you used to do are no longer effective – such as rocking, feeding to sleep and so on.
> - Your baby's naps might be shorter than they were – sometimes just the length of one sleep cycle (35–45 minutes long).
> - You might even find that they have switched to micro naps of 5–10 minutes before startling awake.

Bear in mind that it is normal for babies to wake at night to feed and for some naps to be short. It might also be that they require less daytime sleep than in those early weeks and it is just a case of keeping up with their sleep needs (see page 105). If your baby is having the same daytime naps as they were at two to three months old, it is likely going to have an impact on your nights (in a negative way). It is always worth taking a step back and looking at your baby's day, and considering whether you need to tweak it.

Although this period of sleep development is a permanent change in your baby's sleep architecture and it won't revert to how it used to be, it doesn't mean that you will be stuck in sleep limbo forever!

For some babies (I have noticed particularly those who have

practised independent sleep beforehand), this phase passes quickly and smoothly, and there might not even be any sleep disruption at all. For other babies, the change can be a brutal period of sleep deprivation. These babies will need support and help to get to sleep, and to stay asleep. However, with time and practice you can absolutely get sleep back on track or find a new rhythm with sleep that you haven't had before.

Falling asleep and staying asleep without lots of parental input can be tricky for some babies – especially those with more of a sensitive temperament (more on this on page 146), plus, at around four months, I believe in taking things slowly, to be kind to you and to baby. It isn't a time for any formal 'sleep training', but you don't need to wait it out and do nothing.

Some practical things you can do right now include:

1.  Assess your baby's sleep environment. Is it dark? Is it quiet? Do you need some white noise to drown out snoring, for example? Do you need to stop watching TV in your bedroom at night (or turn on subtitles – a little tip of mine!)? Is your baby appropriately dressed? Are they too hot or too cold? Refer back to the basics we explored in Chapter 4 if you need a refresher.

2.  Assess your baby's routine. I have talked about starting and finishing the day at roughly the same time (see page 102), but at this age you can start to try to aim for naps at roughly similar times and of similar lengths. Making it a little more predictable will help both you and your baby. It doesn't need to be set in stone, but working with your baby and when they need to nap and feed can help everyone.

3.  Think about how your little one falls asleep. You can work on this gradually. On page 108 I talked about practising putting them down – you can continue to play with putting them down awake. I find that the morning nap and bedtime are the

best opportunities to do this. Your baby will be more receptive to a new way of falling asleep.

4. Ask for help. Dealing with sleep deprivation is hard. You can't care for your baby if you don't care for yourself. Get early nights and make sure you have easy-to-prepare meals. If friends or family offer it, accept help. Maybe you can invest in a cleaner, even if it is just occasionally. Perhaps a friend can come and watch the baby so you can get out for some fresh air alone. All the little acts of kindness towards yourself add up throughout the day. Communicate with your partner or other caregivers about how you feel, how you are coping and what you would like to do moving forward. If everyone is on board with what you are doing and how you are feeling it can really help. Drink water, include gentle movement in your day and rest whenever you can.

## HITTING THE MAGIC SIX MONTHS

There is a reason why lots of experts will tell you that you can sleep train at six months. Not only has your baby been alive half of an entire year, but this is when things really move on developmentally. They are far more aware of their environment than previously, they might be rolling (or thinking about it!), they might be sitting up independently and are generally more physically active during the day. Hopefully by six months if your little one has any medical challenges or physical discomfort it has been diagnosed and is being treated. There is a chance your little one might have already dropped night feeds, or might be ready to soon, although this isn't just a simple equation of calories in/calories out. Feeding is more complex than that, and babies feed at night for comfort and connection, not nutrition alone.

There is no rule that you *have* to, or even need to, 'sleep train' at six months. It might be that things are working out really well for you and your baby right now. The thing is, unfortunately, there isn't just some magic switch that flips the day they turn six months. Although you have biology on your side, you might find that it takes work, time and consistency to see an improvement in your little one's sleep. Sleep won't suddenly change overnight, but you have a new opportunity to work on improving things if you want to.

## Looking at your routine

If you don't have a routine by now, you may benefit from introducing one for several reasons. Your little one is capable of sleeping for longer chunks at night, they are starting on solids and they might be moving into their own room. When you move your baby into their own room is really a personal choice, depending on multiple factors, but for some this can be the catalyst to working on sleep.

> The very act of moving baby into their own room sometimes kick-starts parents into action to make a plan.

If you don't have the space available and are room-sharing out of necessity, don't think you can't work on sleep. It is possible to improve sleep while your little one shares a room with you (see page 62).

Sadly, starting solids is also not a magic bullet to better sleep (more on this on page 140) and the very prospect of adding meals to your baby's day can be overwhelming without some sort of structure. Structure is your friend and it doesn't have to be limiting – I actually think knowing when to do things sets you free. You know when baby will be happy to interact with friends, you know when they will want their lunch and you will quickly know if something is wrong.

## Considering sleep training

Lots of people start sleep training at six months, and many consultants advise this, but this doesn't mean that you must rush into anything now. You can still take things slowly, gently and responsively. Choosing a method that suits you, your family and, most of all, your baby is paramount. I outline several different methods in Chapter 8 so that you can weigh up your options.

The idea behind working on sleep is that, once your baby's needs are met (for example, they are fed when needed, nappy changed and healthy), they will hopefully sleep for a solid chunk of time. The aim isn't to ignore them all night – as much as some of the critics would suggest.

It's a common misconception that by teaching your baby to fall asleep independently we are trying to remove their dependence on us – this is far from the case. Our babies are totally dependent on us – to love them, to nurture them and to keep them safe. Sleep training doesn't change this. Solid sleep is a gift – it is not taking anything away from them. We don't want a baby to stop communicating with us – that would be a bizarre, and totally unachievable, goal. I have watched on countless monitors and sat in the rooms of babies who get themselves to sleep. They are not lying there feeling abandoned, they are peacefully sleeping.

We need them to communicate their needs, and those needs don't stop at night-time, but it is about learning to differentiate between when they need us and when they need us to give them the space to get a good night's sleep. Sleep is restorative, it is amazing, we all want it, and need it. I am often told by parents that their baby 'hates sleep'. No one hates sleep; they just haven't learned how to settle for solid periods at night. This is your opportunity to work on this, as slowly and as gently as you like. It is important to choose a method that is right for you and your baby – more on this in the next chapter.

Waiting until six months to start sleep training means that your baby is biologically a better age to potentially sleep for longer periods. From my own practice, I have noticed that babies of six months and over are more receptive to changes in the way they fall asleep and benefit more from a structured routine than younger babies, as well as for all of the reasons I have given previously, such as they are able to stay awake longer in the day, they have solid food to factor into their day, and so on.

It doesn't mean that sleep will be 'perfect' (there is no such thing as perfect sleep) or that there won't be bumps in the road. It is normal for little ones to go through ups and downs with sleep – developmental changes, outside influences, illness and changing sleep requirements all affect sleep. In spite of these things, you should be able to get a solid night's sleep most of the time. It might not be the same as before you had children, but I'll be damned if I am going to let you think that sleep is lost forever now you have become a parent!

It is about learning to differentiate between when babies need us and when they need us to give them the space to get a good night's sleep.

Research tells us that cry-based sleep-training methods are effective. Does this mean they are the best for your baby? Not necessarily. That's why it's important to look at all of your options and see what works for you and your family. Sometimes three to five days of a method that could include tears will solve a sleep problem, but other times it won't. We know that many of the commonly used sleep-training strategies work well if we are consistent. This is why I believe it is important to invest your time in a method that fits well with your baby's temperament and with your belief system and parenting style. I want you to have options.

## Moving your baby into their own room

Safe sleep guidance in the UK is that it is safe to move your baby to their own sleep space *from* six months, but this doesn't mean that you have to. Do not feel pressured to do it sooner than you want to, but equally don't feel guilty if you have been counting down the days until you can move them out.

---

The choice to move your baby into their own room should be yours and yours only.

---

Some babies are quite loud during the night – whether it's moaning, groaning or just wriggling around. This might have been disturbing your sleep and stopping you from getting back to sleep if you wake at night. It can also work the other way round – sometimes we disturb them. It might be that you or your partner snore, or that you disturb baby when you get ready for bed or if you use the toilet at night. I do find that when your little one's sleep cycles mature (see page 30), they become more aware of their environment. For the more sensitive babies, even you turning over in bed can be enough to disturb them if they are in a light sleep. I tend to find this becomes more of an issue as they reach this age, so it may make sense to move them out (if you have a spare room).

Some people see a big improvement in sleep when they move their baby out, while for others it makes no difference, or in fact makes their situation feel harder. As always, do what feels right for you and your baby. You might find that things feel easier if you keep baby in with you or you might just not be ready emotionally for the move, but I generally find that babies adjust well and parents are pleasantly surprised.

Remember, you can still sleep train if you share a room with your baby. You will be using a method where you are in the room with baby or potentially popping in and out of your shared sleep space. Sharing a room doesn't necessarily need to be a barrier to a good night's sleep and, let's not forget, not everyone has the privilege of a spare room.

If you have decided to sleep train and have chosen one of the methods like controlled crying or comforting, it can be easier for baby to be in their own room. If you have chosen habit fading or similar, I think it would be easier to begin in a room that you are sharing with baby.

Some tips for when you do make the move:

1. Don't move them during a time of illness or other disruption (such as starting nursery). Too much change at once can be unsettling. It is all about picking your moment.

2. If they are sleeping in a bedside crib or bed-sharing, you might want to move them into a big cot in your room initially (if you have space). The other option is to keep them in their bedside crib but move it further away from your bed (with the sides up) to get used to being a little further apart first. You could also keep them in their bassinet in their new room before moving them to a cot. Try to use the same positioning in the room if you do that. Or you can just go for it and make a straight switch to a cot.

3. Use slept-in bedding rather than clean bedding when you move baby into their new sleep space so that it smells familiar to them.

4. Stick to your normal bedtime routine, keeping things familiar and in the same order as usual.

5. Make sure their room is set up well and they have appropriate bedding (see Chapter 4). Definitely invest in blackout blinds for those summer months if you can.

6. Consider your baby's temperament (see page 146). You might find that those who have a laid-back temperament find the

transition easy. Those who are more sensitive might need more input from you.

7. You can always change your mind. If it doesn't feel right or your baby hasn't coped well and sleep is worse, you can always bring them back in with you. It's never a failing to change your mind.

It's good to use a baby monitor (see page 61), but if you can already hear baby well from your own room, there is no need to have it on its loudest setting. This means you hear them with an echo, which is particularly unpleasant to wake up to! Also, staring at the baby monitor screen in the dark isn't the best for our own sleep. Use it when you need it, but don't let it become an obsession.

---

If you feel like you are uncomfortable with baby in another room, you can always move them back in with you. You are always allowed to change your mind.

---

### Gradually letting go

*A couple I worked with were nervous about moving their baby out of their bedroom. She was born a little early at 36 weeks and had had some breathing problems. Although these were resolved in the early weeks of her life, it had made her parents quite anxious and they had got into the habit of taking turns to watch her while she slept. Neither of them had felt comfortable moving her into her own room.*

*When I met them, baby Lucy was nearly nine months old. She was sleeping at the end of their bed, in a cot. Her sleep wasn't terrible, but her parents were struggling to relax and switch off. Any little moan, groan or whimper and they were wide awake. They also noticed that*

*Lucy would wake when they went to bed – which varied from around 10 to 11pm. They would give her a feed and put her back into her cot – she was pretty good at getting herself to sleep, but whenever she stirred in the night her parents had a habit of getting her out to check on her. This was disturbing her sleep for sure.*

*We did a lot of work around confidence and pushing their boundaries at night. I challenged them to wait two minutes (with a timer!) before responding to her movements (shuffling or groaning, for example). We then pushed it to five minutes, and then up to ten. They soon realised that Lucy was okay and was settling herself to sleep. Moving Lucy into her own room was a big deal, but they decided that they would likely sleep much better and disturb her far less if she was in her own room. So, they went for it! They used her slept-in bedding and kept their routine as familiar as possible. Lucy surprised them and 'slept through' on the first night. Her parents were still watching her on the monitor for much of those first few nights, but they soon became more relaxed and trusted that she would be okay.*

### Starting solids

Another milestone at this age is starting solids. Working on your little one's sleep really is unrelated to what they eat. There are myths out there that solids will improve sleep or that your little one needs to be a certain weight to sleep through the night, but the evidence tells us otherwise.[1]

Your baby will be ready to start solids at around the six-month mark – the actual age varies for each baby. We should be looking out for the signs of readiness for solid foods, which include:

1. Being able to sit up and hold their head steady.
2. Absence of the 'tongue thrust reflex' – this is when they push food straight back out of their mouth.

**3.** Good enough hand–eye coordination so that they can see food, pick it up and bring it to their mouth.

Frequent night waking, dribbling and looking at your food are *not* signs of readiness. In fact, we can often mistake these signs and introduce solid foods too early, which can potentially wreak havoc with our little one's digestive system, and therefore their sleep! You may find friends and family members suggesting that you 'fill your baby up' so that they will sleep, but this will not help. If anything, it can cause pain, wind and vomiting if your little one overeats. Think about when you have had a big meal – it's unlikely that if you lie down straight away you would have a great night's sleep afterwards. The breast milk or formula that your baby is currently having as their main source of nutrition has all the calories that they need to sleep well – milk will have far more calories than vegetable puree.

It is also a myth that you need to fill babies up with formula – in fact, breast milk and formula have a similar number of calories. If babies are consuming too much formula or cow's milk at night, it can have a real impact on their appetite and therefore the important balance of micronutrients they get from eating solids.

---

At this age, the key to sleep is less about what babies are consuming and more about how they get to sleep, their sleep environment and a good balance of day and night sleep.

---

Babies wake for lots of reasons and it's a common misconception that it is always for hunger. They might need your help getting back to sleep or they might be telling you they are in discomfort or that something else is wrong. Maybe they just need some reassurance, or maybe there is something else going on.

**SAFETY FIRST**

There is some outdated, and sometimes dangerous, advice out there about adding porridge or rusks to bottles. Not only will this not help with sleep, but it's also a choking risk. The only thing you should be giving your little one in a bottle is formula or expressed breast milk, and this should be supervised by you.

Don't give your little one a bottle to drink on their own in their cot – this poses a risk of choking, aspiration and, not to forget, tooth decay. It can also cause your little one to be reliant on milk to get to sleep and to stay asleep. This means you could find yourself replacing their bottle of milk between each sleep cycle in the night.

## ROUTINE

I have talked about the importance of routine, but I believe that at this age you can work towards it being even more predictable. It is still important to have some flexibility, but having something that you and your baby can rely on will really help you. Remember what I have already spoken about – starting the day at roughly the same time each day, and bedtime routine. These two things are the foundation of your routine.

If you haven't already, this is a good time to get your little one to bed a bit earlier. I do find that a bedtime between 6.30 and 8pm works best for babies of four to six months. If you have a 'low sleep needs' baby (see below) and they wake early in the morning, closer to 8pm might suit you best.

It is important to keep on top of your little one's changing sleep needs – this period between four and six months is a short stage in their lives, but their day could look vastly different at four months to when they are six months, and also differ from baby to baby. Some parents fall into the trap of expecting their baby to need the same amount of sleep as when they were smaller, which results in nap battles and generally a miserable time of it.

---

We don't want our babies to become overtired, but under-tiredness really is a routine killer.

---

Observe your baby and experiment with naps to get your day balanced well. Most little ones at this age are still on three naps, but occasionally some six-month-olds will be moving towards two naps. They are all different, so judge it on your baby and, if it works, it works!

There is no such thing as a perfect routine, but many babies this age benefit from a long nap after their lunch. You can try aiming for this and seeing if it works for your baby. If you have a baby who struggles to wind down for naptime, you can introduce a 'mini' bedtime routine – this allows your baby a chance to slow down, relax and lets them know what is coming. Babies love predictability!

Of course, it is always important to look at our babies for the answer if we are unsure whether they are getting enough sleep. Have a think about the following signs:

**1.** Your baby has periods of time during the day where they are happy, alert and content.
**2.** Your baby is hitting their developmental milestones (pretty much – these also vary!). If you are ever unsure about this, do consult your doctor or health visiting team if you are in the UK.
**3.** What you are doing with naps and bedtimes seems to be working. If it ain't broke, don't fix it!

> **YOUR BABY'S SLEEP NEEDS**
>
> While we can talk about average amounts of sleep and naps, there are always babies who sit outside of these parameters. You will know if you have a 'low sleep needs' baby as they will tend to sleep a lot less than their peers and be happy, content and thriving. They might take short naps and drop their naps much faster than the norm. On the flip side, a 'high sleep needs' baby will sleep much more than their contemporaries, possibly for a longer period overnight, with more frequent and longer naps than most their age. They will also take longer to drop their naps. Adults are the same — some adults are happy on seven hours' sleep per night, and others need nine.

## MOVING FORWARD

So, you have decided you want to work on sleep, your baby is now at the right age to do so and the timing feels right for your family. How do we do this? How do we choose where to start? How do we know what feels right for us and our babies? What does the evidence say about what is safe and what isn't? I know so many of you will have concerns about crying, and that is what I am going to cover for you next.

### Nurturing your baby through their cries

It may be that you don't want to attempt any sleep-training method that will involve your baby crying, and that's okay, but I would encourage you to reread the crying section on page 39 and the following section to help you reflect on your attitude to crying.

One of the classic falsehoods about 'sleep training' is that we teach our babies to stop communicating with us. Of course, it is vital for our babies to communicate with us, so the aim of sleep training is never to stop them communicating or to stop them crying – or even to make them cry. It is about nurturing them through crying at bedtime and enabling them to have a restful night's sleep. I have never met a family who stopped their baby from communicating with them because of improving their sleep. Many families have reported that they know quickly when something is wrong at night, because their babies normally sleep so soundly. It becomes very obvious when a baby who sleeps well ordinarily is poorly.

There are strategies available to hold space for crying, to tune in and ask ourselves what our little ones need from us, and to have the opportunity to co-regulate, by which I mean be present and help them regulate their crying. It is important to be honest – if you are changing the way your little one falls asleep, there is likely going to be some crying. This is your baby communicating to you that things feel different and that they don't like change. Tears at bedtime can feel difficult, but that doesn't mean that you are doing anything wrong.

---

If our children are learning to walk and they stumble and cry, we don't immediately tell them to give up and never try to walk again, so why do we do this at bedtime?

---

Crying can feel painful for us, but there are reasons why it can often feel worse than it is.

A common question I get asked by parents is, 'How long will my baby cry for when I am changing how they fall asleep?' The answer is, 'I don't know.' They might not cry at all, they might cry for a few minutes, or it could be longer. We really don't know until we try. If it feels like the crying is too much or it doesn't feel like you are getting anywhere, it is always okay to change how you are doing things.

If your little one is crying excessively, I would have a think about these things before you continue:

1. Is my baby well?
2. Is there anything bothering my baby? Do they have a dirty nappy? Are they too hot or too cold?
3. Is my baby tired enough for bed? (If sleep pressure – see page 29 – has not built up enough, they can cry far more.)
4. Is the method I am currently doing best suited to my baby? It might be that you change method – either to a more 'hands-off' approach if it feels like you are overstimulating them or to a more gradual gentle approach if your little one is sensitive to the changes you are making. Also consider their temperament (see below).
5. Have they had a good balance of day sleep ahead of their night?
6. Are they hungry?
7. Are they overtired?

If we take all these things into account then, while we absolutely cannot eliminate crying for all of the reasons above, we can minimise crying during the process.

### Considering your baby's temperament

You know your baby best, but have you ever thought about what sort of temperament they have? Are they laid back? Do they need a lot of comforting in new situations? Are they fairly flexible and easy-going? Or are they easily upset?

Dr W. Thomas Boyce, professor of paediatrics and psychiatry, and author of *The Orchid and the Dandelion*, explains this in more detail.[2] He talks about two types of children: the 'orchids' and the 'dandelions'. He says that around 80 per cent of children are 'dandelions', who thrive in most environments and are resilient. He also talks about the other 20 per cent who are 'orchids', who tend to be more sensitive and need particular conditions to thrive (just as the flower does).

I really like the analogy of these flowers. It's a useful way to think about your baby and their temperament. You might be wondering how you know if you have an 'orchid' child. Well, if you have one you probably already know, you just haven't put a label on it yet. Orchids need a lot more contact from their parents and are more sensitive to lights, sounds, smells and their environment. They might have been labelled as clingy or fussy. They often need more help to get to sleep at bedtime, wake frequently and need very specific conditions to sleep well. Having an 'orchid' doesn't mean that all hope is lost though – it just means that you need to work a bit more carefully, over a longer period, with a gradual sleep plan. With the right care, 'orchids', just like their flower, can flourish (and get a good night's sleep!).

As your baby grows, you will get to know their personality and their likes and dislikes. Some babies like to be patted; some like to be stroked. Some like to be sung to; some like white noise. Some don't like any of these things. Some are receptive to touch, while for some it makes them agitated.

Working out your little one's preferences, along with their temperament, is the first clue to how you might approach a sleep plan.

## ATTACHMENT CONCERNS

Some parents are scared into inaction due to false claims about sleep training and attachment. There has been a lot of awareness around attachment in recent years, which is a positive thing for parenting and for our children. However, alongside this has come a lot of anxiety – some parents are now crippled with fear that, if their child is unhappy for even a moment, they will have damaged their attachment. We know from research that crying in itself does not damage attachment. If your little one is crying and you comfort them, this is not going to damage attachment. If you leave them for a short period of time, this is not going to damage attachment. Even if you sleep train, it is not going to damage attachment.[3]

Research from Harvard University has shown that small lapses in attention in a loving and responsive environment cause no need for concern. In fact, research tells us that being responsive 50 per cent of the time, leads to secure attachment in the long term.[4] The way we parent our babies is important – we want to ensure that we develop a secure base for them to return to. We want them to know we are always here, but that it is okay to explore the world and, if they get upset, we will still be here. I would hazard a guess that if you are the type of parent reading this book, it is likely that you are incredibly responsive and your baby is well attached to you. Not everyone has the privilege, or the capacity, to respond to their babies at every single moment. That is not realistic. There will be times when they are crying in the car, when we are attending to their siblings, when the dinner is about to burn, when we need to go to work or when we just need to put them down in a safe space.

---

You don't have to choose between attachment and sleep. You can, in fact, be an 'attachment parent' and sleep train if you want to.

---

In fact, by getting a better night's sleep you may improve your attachment; if you are well-slept, you are happier and far more likely to engage positively and play and bond with your baby during the day. This in turn means that baby is happier. Your baby knows that you will meet their needs. Leaving the room for a brief period (if this is a method you choose to do) is not going to damage your attachment. Babies are not attached all day long and suddenly traumatised at bedtime.

### ATTACHMENT PARENTING

You may have heard of attachment parenting and be wondering what it is. It's a philosophy of parenting made popular by Dr William and nurse Martha Sears in their 1993 book *The Baby Book*. The theory is that you maximise closeness and responsiveness when you parent – you bedshare, breastfeed on demand and answer any upset immediately. There has been much debate on the topic over the years, and the research has shown that attachment parenting is no better or worse than other parenting styles – so, you don't have to bed-share or babywear to have good attachment! It is not scientifically linked to more 'secure attachment'.

Attachment theory is all about helping your baby to learn and process new feelings and experiences, while supporting them. We support them during the day to learn about the world, and the same applies at night-time. We can support them to get a better night's sleep so that they can be happy and thrive during the daytime. You can maintain a great attachment and get a good night's sleep! You do not have to choose. It is possible to nurture independent sleep, while still being emotionally available to your baby.

Unfortunately, negative press sticks around for a long time. During the 1980s there was a terrible situation in Romania where thousands of babies were left in orphanages (this was due to restrictive reproductive health policies at the time – women under 40 had no access to abortions and there was a ban on contraception). These babies and children were abused, neglected and had almost no adult contact for much of their daily lives. They stopped crying because they knew no one was ever going to come to them. It's abhorrent to even think about and the details are incredibly harrowing. So why am I talking about this? Well, researchers looked at these children and noticed that their attachment was severely impacted (this is not a surprise to anyone who has read about how they were treated). Unfortunately, this research has been used as the base of an argument against all crying strategies and is still referred to some 40 years later.

Now, in the modern world, in a loving home, with an attached baby and caregiver, who is responsive and loving, it is utterly incomparable. These poor babies were left for months on end, not moments. Anyone who is reading this book will be here because they want to do the best for their baby and their family. You will be looking at the strategies available where you can hold space for your little one's crying, not to simply ignore it – or neglect them for months on end. Our babies know we are going to come back.

One of the key findings that I have noticed in my practice over the years is that attachment seems to improve in many senses after improving sleep. This is also reflected in the research where maternal mood was reported to improve. An Australian study showed that the mothers of sleep-trained babies were less depressed and more likely to be in better physical health.[5]

One study in Sweden looked at 95 families, who used a version of 'cry it out'.[6] They studied the behaviour of the infants during the day and found that their security and attachment had increased as a result of the sleep intervention. It also found that their 'behaviour' and eating had improved. Of course, we always need to be objective about the research, but it seems to be overwhelmingly positive. I firmly believe that looking at your own baby and what works for them is the most important thing. We could debate all day long about the topic, but, when it comes to the crux, we just want better sleep, for us and our babies. What we do know is that outcomes are, on the whole, positive and that sleep interventions can be effective when done in the right way for the family, and the baby.[7]

I truly believe that if babies were traumatised, damaged and neglected they would continue to be so all of the time. It makes no sense to me that they would be happy, well-attached and thriving during the day, and suddenly become traumatised at bedtime. So, your baby who is happy all day, signals for you to pick them up, laughs when you blow a raspberry, rests their head on your shoulder when they are tired, is not suddenly unattached when you put them to bed.

### Your resilient baby

D.W. Winnicott, a paediatrician and child psychotherapist, created the term the 'good-enough mother'.[8] He reminds us that our children can manage our flaws and imperfections. That they are able to adapt to their situation, the parent–child relationship and any changes that we present to them – and that includes new ways of falling asleep. It doesn't mean we are failing if we find the process difficult. Let's not forget that you are probably tired and this makes it far harder to face a new challenge, whether that is changing how you do things or coping with your baby's tears.

We can only do our level best to support our babies and children as they grow. Not all families are suited to sleep training, which is why it is so important to be kind to yourself in the process and be prepared to change things up if you need to.

There is a misunderstanding that all sleep training refers to the 'cry it out' method (which I don't practise myself, although I will cover it later), but it is far more nuanced than this with many different options. Sometimes it may be something as simple as the introduction of a regular bedtime routine, if you haven't got that in place already, or a tweak to naps, for example. It is important not to underestimate the power of a well-balanced, predictable day and evening routine. In the next chapter, I start by outlining several ways to set up things for a settled bedtime that don't involve any particular sleep methods.

However, whether you can cope with some tears or prefer no tears at all, there are lots of ways you can work on sleep. I'll go on to give you clear guidance on several sleep methods, so you can make an informed choice and work out which feel best for your family – don't expect to know the answer to this before you start. It's not always clear-cut. Sometimes we need to try things first to see how they go. As I have said many times, you can always change your mind.

# 8

# WORKING ON YOUR BABY'S SLEEP

Sometimes it can feel like the Wild West out there, with so many different voices, ideas and statements about what is the right or wrong way to deal with a baby's sleep. What works for one family might not work for another – I want to help you find what works for you.

In this chapter I am going to outline different ways to work on your baby's sleep, so you can make an informed choice about what you do (or don't do) next. I tell you the different names and terms for each approach, but my aim is to cut through the jargon and explain how each one works so that you can try it out for yourself if you wish to. It is all about challenging yourself and your baby's boundaries, while making sure that you don't feel overwhelmed.

I start with the very gentlest way to work on sleep, and finish with the 'strictest'. There is no secret sauce to sleep – instead, it's about matching up the right method to your family. You are allowed to change your mind and to change tack. You can also make up your own method. You might take some parts from one and other parts from another. You might look at them all and think, 'Gosh none of these are for me!' And you know what? That's okay – you don't *have* to do anything. It can feel really overwhelming to even think about it all (ironically, when we are sleep-deprived it can be even harder to think about!).

Some parents get lucky and have a baby who seemingly 'sleeps through the night' with very little work or input, while others seem to work on sleep for weeks or months and make slow progress. Although we have different beliefs as parents and our little ones are all different – in their temperament and their history – I have included some common techniques that I know have worked well for many babies.

To see changes in how your baby sleeps, you need to change how you do things, even if it's just little tweaks. There are some methods that I personally prefer, having seen results with my own children and in my practice over the years. Most of the methods that I'm going to mention here assume that your baby is between six and twelve months at this point. I don't generally advise 'sleep training' for babies under the age of six months, though the exceptions are the 'fade it out' method (see page 173), which is suitable for three to six months and a quick 'pause', as I described earlier in the book (see page 110), where you literally pause for a moment before going to comfort your baby.

---

**CHECKING FOR UNDERLYING PROBLEMS**

If you are introducing a new way of falling asleep, first of all make sure your little one is comfortable, content and in good health. If your baby has an allergy, medical condition or bodily tension that is causing discomfort, it is going to be hard to work on sleep. If you have a nagging feeling that something is up, always get it checked out by a professional. Parental instinct is strong and shouldn't be ignored, but we should also not over-medicalise things if we don't need to.

---

There are a few bits of housekeeping to think about before you get started on a method, which is up next.

## BABY COMFORTERS

You may have been given a small toy or soft blanket as a baby gift or you might be considering buying one for your baby to provide a sense of safety and security. As well as 'comforters', these are called 'transitional objects' or sometimes a 'lovey'.

I really like comforters, especially if you want to move towards having a baby who can settle themselves at bedtime. Their comforter is a great signal to your little one when it is time to switch off and relax at bedtime or naptime. They can also be super useful when starting childcare, going on holiday or being in a strange environment, especially when that means sleeping elsewhere. They smell and feel familiar and are, literally, comforting.

At around six months old, your baby will go through a cognitive change, where they realise they are no longer part of you. It is this moment when they begin to form their own sense of identity and independence. It is also when you might notice separation anxiety. This can be a really good time to introduce a comforter. Not all babies will take to one – I have seen many over the years who just ignore them, as much as their parents might try. However, if you are consistent and keep offering one at sleep times, many little ones will become attached and begin to use their comforter to get to sleep and to help them back to sleep when they wake during the night. They can also be a good tool when trying to ditch the dummy.

If you want to introduce a comforter, make sure it doesn't have long fur, loose eyes or buttons and isn't so big it could get wrapped around your baby. The Lullaby Trust advises that babies should sleep in a completely clear cot until 12 months. This means that if you are using one before this age, you should take the comforter out once your baby is asleep. It is often a confusing topic for parents, as there are comforters on the market that are breathable. I believe we should make our own informed choices on this subject (and all parenting subjects!).

Some tips for using a comforter:

- You could start from six months old.
- Stick to one that is ideally washable, and make sure you have a spare.
- Sleep with it overnight or wear it down your top for a bit so it smells of you (if you are breastfeeding you can even put a bit of breast milk on it!).
- Don't worry if your little one doesn't take to it straight away. As with most of what I talk about, it's just something to have in your toolbox – it is not an essential item.

**Safety first:** safe sleep guidance is to remove comforters once your baby is asleep until the age of 12 months.

## DEVELOPMENTAL CONSIDERATIONS

While we are talking about a fairly small age range (six to twelve months), a lot of things happen developmentally during this time. Some babies will be rolling, some sitting up and some standing. These things all need to be considered when it comes to choosing a sleep method. As I mentioned earlier, once your baby can roll both ways, you can allow them to find a comfortable sleeping position. This might mean that they are trying to settle on their front, for example, and that, when you are reassuring them, you are doing this with your hand on their back. It could also be on their side or you could be patting their bottom too! It depends on what your little one likes and responds well to. You sometimes need to think outside of the box, depending on what you are presented with.

Your little one might sit up as soon as you put them into their cot. The key here is to make sure they are definitely ready for sleep. Bedtime is the best time to start any new changes, as you have biology on your side – sleep pressure is high and your little one really wants to go to sleep, I promise. Sometimes it can help if you nudge bedtime just that little bit later.

Don't panic if they sit up – it's normal for them to want to practise this skill in their cot. If your baby isn't upset, I'd 100 per cent leave them to it. You only need to comfort or reassure them if they are asking for your help. Once you have chosen your sleep method, you can practise this regardless of whether they are sitting up or not. I promise they will lie down eventually!

The same goes for standing in the cot. Don't turn it into a battle or a game. If you keep trying to lie them down over and over again, they will either laugh and think it's silly, or they will get upset, frustrated and potentially overstimulated. I tend to advise gently lying them down once or twice, but any more than that and you are heading into tricky territory.

---

One thing I do find helpful is to tap the mattress – it can be a signal for them to sit or lie down. It doesn't always work though! It's about experimenting and seeing what your baby responds to.

---

### WHEN TO MAKE A CHANGE: NAPS OR NIGHT-TIME?

Some families go all out and stick to one settling method for all sleeps straight away. Others will start at bedtime initially and go from there. Others will solely work on bedtime and night-time, and then naps later. It really depends on your baby and how receptive they are to change. If naps feel difficult to navigate, perhaps choose one nap per day to work on initially and then gradually introduce the change to other naps.

## SLEEP METHODS AND FEEDING

By the age of six months, you may have developed a bit of a rhythm with your baby's feeds, especially if they are eating solids. Some babies will be on just three to four milk feeds across twenty-four hours, and some will be on a lot more than that! Feeding is so personal and individual, I would never tell you that you can't feed your baby or that they don't need a feed. Many babies feed to sleep and sleep fine, but lots of them don't. Lots of parents find that their babies wake very frequently and need to be fed back to sleep again. If this isn't a problem for you and it feels okay, it's absolutely fine to continue doing what you are doing. However, if your situation feels unsustainable and you want to improve things, working away from feeding to sleep will likely help your situation.

So, when do we give a feed and when don't we? It's all down to a bit of experimentation. If your baby wakes up soon after they last fed, you can try the sleep methods in this chapter and see if they settle. If it's much later in the night and you think they might be hungry, you can go ahead and feed them. The key is pushing the boundaries and attempting to settle instead of feeding when you feel comfortable doing so. They might just surprise you!

If you choose a stricter method, you can still decide to do a feed or two in the night – you won't ruin things if you do this. As with anything, you can always change your mind either way, even at the very last moment. I never want you to feel like you are sticking to a rule that feels like you have failed if you bend it.

---

If your situation feels unsustainable and you want to improve things, working away from feeding to sleep will likely help your situation.

---

## TEETHING

Teething is a valid barrier to sleep, but also gets a really bad rap. When your little one is cutting a tooth, it could certainly hinder your progress with sleep or you might get some disrupted nights, but it's not as clear-cut as this. I genuinely believe that teething is not a reason to avoid working on sleep altogether. I have heard so many times across the years from parents who claim their little one has been 'teething for months'.

Teething is most likely to affect your little one's sleep while the tooth is actually cutting through the gum. It can obviously be uncomfortable, but it is a normal, natural process that all infants go through. As with all these things, it will affect some more than others. For some babies, their teeth will emerge with no disturbance at all – honestly. For others, it will be obvious when they are teething, and can be a struggle. Here are some common things to look out for:

1. You might be able to see a red and sore bit of gum where the tooth is emerging.
2. Your baby will likely have a red cheek, which tends to be on the side where the tooth will sit.
3. They might rub their cheek or their ear – jaw pain often refers up to our ears (if you are unsure, you can always get your GP to check their ears in case it's actually an ear infection).
4. There will probably be quite a bit of drooling – although this is common for babies anyway as they are not able to hang on to the saliva in their mouths like we can. You might find their saliva ramps up a bit in the approach to being ready for solid foods too. This is the body's way of preparing them to be able to break down and eat solid foods.
5. They might bite things – or you. Although, again, chewing things and putting things in their mouths is normal baby

behaviour. It can soothe sore gums, but it is also how they explore the world.

6. They might just generally seem a bit unhappy or irritable. This goes for all of us when we have toothache, I think!

7. You might notice that, if they are at an age when they eat solids, they go off their food or seem fussier with it. It is not that fun eating with a sore tooth. Continue to offer food as normal, and you might want to consider sticking mostly to foods you know they like. Cool things like yoghurt, cucumber (grated or peeled) and watermelon are popular with teething babies.

8. It's possible you might see a disturbance in their sleep – they might take longer to settle, seem fretful during their sleep or start waking early in the morning.

What teething doesn't do is transform sleep entirely. If you are pretty much on track, it honestly will not completely derail how your little one settles – this will only happen if we move our boundaries so far that they forget how they used to go to sleep. For example, if you start co-sleeping, your little one will very quickly learn that these are the conditions under which they fall asleep. If you are okay with that (or whatever you are doing), it's always okay, but if it's something you don't want to start doing, you must stay steadfast and not do it! Sounds simple, right? I know this is hard in practice – more on this later!

When a tooth is cutting, you might need to offer your little one a bit more support than usual during the night (think cuddles or feeds, depending on what they like!), but I don't believe we should blame long-term sleep challenges on teething. In theory, the disruption should be short-lived, even if they get a couple of teeth in quick succession. As a rule, I'd say it takes around three to seven days on average for a tooth to cut. If your issues have been going on for weeks or months, it is probably not down to teething. After all, your baby is going to be teething for a few years in total!

Some things you can do to help with teething:

1. There are lots of teething toys on the market that can help. You can also try chilling them in the fridge – don't put anything frozen in your baby's mouth.

2. Cool drinks of water or cold foods can help (don't cool down formula, just give this at its regular or room temperature).

3. You could consider giving your baby over-the-counter pain medication. I don't advise doing this 'just in case', as I have known a worrying number of families tell me they've given pain relief for weeks on end. Pain medications will not improve sleep unless baby is in pain. If you are unsure, please speak to your pharmacist or doctor.

4. Your baby might feed more when they are teething – this is fine. This can be due to excess fluid loss due to drooling, but often it's just for comfort (which is okay if it is okay with you!).

5. I am a big fan of baby massage for teething – some gentle circles on each side around the jaw and some sweeping strokes down the outside of the jaw can help.

## THE DUMMY

If you are going to be working on your baby's sleep, you might want to consider whether or not the dummy is serving you and your baby. Getting rid of it can be done in conjunction with the sleep changes and methods below if that works for your family. If you would like to do this more gradually, you could get rid of the dummy before sleep training, or afterwards – whatever works best for your baby and their temperament.

If you are working on a sleep method and you are keeping the dummy, you might need to be prepared to replace the dummy for your baby at regular intervals, unless they are on the older end of the age range and are able to replace it themselves. I advise putting extras in the cot to give them the best chance of finding it.

The NHS guidance if you are in the UK is to stop giving your baby a dummy somewhere between six and twelve months, so the timing is right if you are thinking about getting rid of it now. You can try initially taking the dummy out of your baby's mouth just before they fall asleep to get them used to the feeling, but it tends to be a quicker (and I think fairer) process if you just go for it.

Unfortunately, there isn't some fancy solution to ditching the dummy– cold turkey is the most effective way. I tend to advise first limiting dummies to sleep times only (this is really what we should be doing anyway!) and then taking away the dummy for the first time at bedtime. This is when you have biology on your side. Remember I talked about how your baby is most likely to accept a new way of falling asleep at bedtime? Well, this is the case for the removal of the dummy too. Once you decide to get rid of it, you'll need to stick to your guns though. It is likely that your little one could get upset, but continue to comfort them with whatever you usually do – rocking, swaying, patting, cuddling – and I promise that they will forget all about it eventually!

If you are struggling, you can try removing the dummy just before your baby falls asleep. This can be a good way to get them used to the feeling of falling asleep without it.

## SETTING UP FOR SUCCESS

Before you even begin considering introducing any new way of changing how your baby sleeps, there are things you can put in place to improve your chances of success.

### Keeping the calm

An important precursor to settling to sleep – for all of us, adults included – is how we feel in ourselves. If we are calm, our nervous system relaxes and we find it easier to go to sleep. If you are changing how your baby falls asleep, it is very possible that they are not going to seem very calm. If your baby is agitated at bedtime (or any other sleep time), then refocusing on helping them to relax, rather than to sleep, can transform how their bedtime goes. Once your little one is really agitated, it can take a while for them to calm down, so if you can instil some calm before you get to that place it can really help.

To do this, first focus on your own state of mind. If you are stressed, anxious and worked up about putting your baby to bed, they will pick up on it. Try some deep breathing and you can even say out loud, 'Everything is going to be fine. We *will* go to sleep eventually, and everything is okay. I am safe, I love my baby, we are okay.'

Once you have gathered yourself, even if you step away from your baby for 30 seconds to do this (make sure they are in a safe space), you will approach things in a calmer way. I am not saying this is easy. I know these times can feel desperate, but you need to try to stay calm for your baby.

> If you are finding it hard to calm down, I would enlist the help of your partner or close friend or family member to help you. Perhaps they could give the bedtime settling a go? Maybe you could get out for a ten-minute walk and return to take over.

Once you feel more centred, next up it is time to help your baby to relax too. If you haven't already, work on establishing an effective bedtime routine (see page 105), then add to that with a lullaby, a cuddle, rocking them a little in your arms as you sing, reading a bedtime story, giving them a massage . . . the list goes on. Remember, babies are all different so find different things relaxing. My oldest loved me singing to her before bed – she would instantly relax in my arms. My middle and youngest would have wriggled out of my arms before I could finish the first verse (don't take offence if your baby doesn't like your singing!). My middle child loved a massage before bed, and my youngest just loves a quick cuddle and straight into his cot.

So, if you do nothing else, think about how you can help your baby to calm down. Try different ways until you find what works and in a way that is compatible with the methods you are using to change how they fall asleep. As always, if a way of calming your baby doesn't work or stops working at any point, change it.

### Soothing phrases and songs

Babies and children love repetition, familiarity and your voice especially. So try choosing a sentence or phrase to use at each bedtime or naptime. You could sing a short song or stick to a simple phrase.

Some examples include:

- 'Night night, sleep tight, see you in the morning.'
- 'Love you to the moon and back.'
- 'Sleepy time now, love you.'
- 'Night night, ssh ssh.'

When my youngest was a small baby, I sang Bob Marley's 'Three Little Birds'. It calmed us both down if things ever got fractious at bedtime. (Anecdotally, many parents report that reggae music has a particularly calming effect on their babies, and them!)

Your phrase or song can be absolutely anything – whatever comes to mind. You will say this at each bedtime and naptime – don't be surprised if eventually your little one says it back to you. I have lost count of the number of times that old clients have said this to me! It can be very sweet to finally get that communication back. It is never a waste of time.

## Choosing the right time

To give yourself the best chance of a new sleep method working, you need to allocate time and space to work on it. It's not a good time to do it if you are about to go on holiday, your little one is about to start nursery or they are poorly. Also, if you have lots going on socially – if you have a family party, wedding or other events in quick succession – it could scupper your plans. This does *not* mean you can't have a life or get out of the home while working on sleep, but you need to be able to provide the opportunity for your little one to sleep when they are tired, and if they are practising settling asleep independently, they need to have their safe sleep space.

We all have busy lives and, let's face it, there is a never a perfect time to start – but there will be better times than others. I often say a Friday can work well (if you don't work weekends), as you can have time to rest and recuperate at the weekend, and potentially share the load with a partner. Depending on which method you choose, you might make really great progress in just a few days, so don't feel like you need to block out months in your social calendar.

**Please note:** in the approaches I've outlined below, I've given an example of the number of nights for each method. Bear in mind that they could take more or less time than stated.

---

### MEETING YOUR BABY'S NEEDS

Try to ensure you are meeting all your baby's needs before you start trying to introduce a new way of sleeping:

- Have some nice connection time before bed (your undivided attention, lots of cuddles).

---

- Make sure they are well-fed.
- Make sure they are comfortable, that they have a clean nappy and that they are ready for bed.

## UNDERSTANDING WHAT SUCCESS MEANS FOR YOU

Each family will have a different goal in mind when it comes to working on sleep. You might want your baby to sleep for a long chunk at night, to sleep all night with little intervention or it might just be that you want to be able to settle them a bit quicker when they wake in the night, or be able to put them down in their cot in the evenings so you can have some time to yourself.

Some families choose to simply work on routine tweaks and managing their own sleep as a starting point. It might be that you need to sit down with your partner and redistribute the balance of care for your baby, the household chores or how you can get in a nap during the day. It might be that you still rock or feed your baby to sleep, but work on some more regular timings (see page 102). This might be all you need as a family.

You may also need more than this. You might find yourself in the depths of a sleep deprivation crisis and need to totally transform the way your baby sleeps, and this is okay too.

---

We only need to change things if they aren't working for us, and if they aren't working then don't feel guilty about needing to change things.

---

You might also want to change things but be afraid of it not working. Fear of failure can be a big roadblock for many parents. If it all feels like it's too much, then you can make small, manageable changes.

## *An unsustainable routine*

*I worked with a family of two dads and their baby girl Gracie, who was seven months old. She had been sleeping really well until they went on holiday to the US and she was jetlagged when they got home. Her parents were in the habit of rocking her to sleep and, before long, they were taking it in turns to rock her throughout the night (six to eight times!). Phil was an engineer and started really struggling to focus at work, so David had begun to take on more of the night wakings. What had felt like an 'easy' way to get Gracie to sleep had become a really unpleasant and unsustainable approach for their family. David had started to feel incredibly guilty — he admitted to me that he felt like he was failing Gracie, and failing Phil. They had gone through a lot to have Gracie in their lives and he wanted her to be getting the very best start in life. He also couldn't face the idea of letting her cry.*

*We worked through all of the background info — how they got to this point — and exactly what was going on with Gracie's sleep. The first point of action that we started with was optimising her sleep environment. She was starting the day very early (after a very broken night) and would not settle easily come 5am. The first thing we did was properly blackout their bedroom (she was still room-sharing). We also added some white noise (to drown out Phil's snoring!).*

*The next thing was routine tweaks. They were attempting a bedtime with a very late third nap — I explained that Gracie wasn't actually tired enough for bed, especially as she was doing a long lunchtime nap (normally in her pram) of around two hours. A nap at almost 6pm and trying to get her down for 7.30pm was never going to happen, hence why they were rocking her for almost an hour. I said they needed to either cut the nap or push bedtime later. We cut the nap. This meant that, although she was a little fussy come bath time, she was actually ready for bed. They were able to rock her for only ten minutes and she went off to sleep. Even this small change had an immediate effect of making bedtime easier and reducing her night wakings by almost half – she woke four times that first night. They rocked her back to sleep as usual.*

*The next step was moving on to intermittent rocking. So, they would rock her for 30 seconds, then stop for 30 seconds and be still. The time when they were still would increase, so that eventually she was held to sleep. Then she was put down sleepy (but awake) with their hands on her chest. She did whimper a little, but no full-blown crying at all.*

*When we finished our support, she was waking one to two times per night, but they were okay with that. They were relieved that she could go to bed far more quickly, wake less often and they didn't need to force that third nap that she didn't need anymore. We are still in touch to this day, and Gracie is a happy, healthy three-year-old who sleeps through the night.*

## MAKING EYE CONTACT

It's a very old-fashioned approach to say you can't make eye contact when you are working on sleep. It's *always* okay to give your baby eye contact. Some babies need that reassurance from you to relax and go to sleep. Some parents tell me that they prefer to avert their gaze a little, otherwise their babies want to play, but, overall, I wouldn't worry about it! If it feels right in the moment, you can absolutely look your baby in the eye. If you find it over-stimulating for them, you can avert your gaze if you prefer. It's unlikely to have a huge impact either way, so try not to overthink it.

## THE SLEEP STAIRCASE

Taking your first steps to making changes can feel daunting – I like to think of it like a high staircase. It looks overwhelming at the start, but, once you get started, it's easier to climb than you think. And I want you to go at your own pace, the pace that is right for you and your baby, while respecting your parental style and views.

You might find that you are happy at step 1, 2 or 3 and you just stay there. You don't necessarily need to reach the top. You might take weeks, or even months to get there. However, you or your baby might surprise you and head to the top in a matter of days.

This is an example of what your sleep staircase might look like – it will be different for everyone, depending on your starting point and your end goal:

- Step 1: feeding, rocking, patting, bouncing, cuddling to sleep (these are examples of what you might be doing already, insert others here!).
- Step 2: feeding, rocking, patting, bouncing, cuddling *almost* to sleep.
- Step 3: baby falling asleep in their cot with you patting, singing, reassuring from the side.
- Step 4: baby *almost* falling asleep with you patting, singing, reassuring (but you leave!).
- Step 5: some short verbal or physical reassurance before they go to sleep (your sleep phrase or a quick kiss or pat).
- Step 6: being able to say your sleep phrase and leaving baby to settle themselves.

In order to move up the ladder, we need to change how we are doing things. This is where different sleep methods come in. Whichever method you choose, the idea is that you move up the staircase – at your own pace.

## WAIT IT OUT

Before we get into the really proactive methods, I wanted to mention the option to simply wait it out. Even if you do absolutely nothing with your baby's sleep, there will still come a day when they get a settled night's sleep or 'sleep through the night'. All humans are different, just as all children are different. This means that it could happen at any time, or it might not happen until later in childhood. It is always okay if, for example, you choose to bed-share or sit with your child until they fall asleep for as long as it works for you and your family. You only need to change things if it is not sustainable or is no longer working for your family.

Waiting it out is a valid option for many. Sometimes we just want the permission to do nothing other than get through the days and the nights and relax about it.

You might feel you 'should' be changing things under the duress of others, when in actual fact you are okay with how things are. It can feel empowering to make the choice to wait it out.

## BED-SHARING

This is not a suggestion you will often hear from sleep consultants, but, for some people, bed-sharing with their baby is a lifesaver. If you are someone who gets up to breastfeed your baby multiple times per night, you might just find that this means you can rest while feeding and get more sleep than if your baby was sleeping separately, as you can simply roll them onto their back after feeding (always make sure you are following safe co-sleeping guidance – see page 51). Some people just don't have the energy, patience or motivation to attempt to tend to their baby sleeping in another sleep space. They might also just really enjoy it, and that's okay too! You must always follow safe bed-sharing advice – see page 53.

Bed-sharing can be a simple fix and a pleasurable experience for those who like it. If you are able to sleep through your little one's stirrings, you might get more sleep than sleeping separately. Bear in mind that if you are a light sleeper, bed-sharing could mean less sleep overall. The downside is that it can be tricky when siblings arrive, can sometimes cause conflict with a partner and, for some, it can become tricky when baby is on the move. Some families find that a mattress on the floor is safer than an average bed once their baby is on the move. If you bed-share and you are happy, then you don't need to feel guilty. So many people keep it a secret, but there's really no shame in it.

---

People across the world share beds with their babies – we just need to use our knowledge of safer sleep guidelines to keep our babies safe while we do it.

---

## THE TRANSFER

Some babies feed or are rocked to sleep (or however else you might 'get' them to sleep) and then are able to sleep soundly throughout the night. If you want to hold your baby in any of these ways to get them to sleep, you need to know how to transfer them to their cot, which might also give you a few hours in the evening without your baby sleeping on you.

So how do you do it?

**1.** The most important thing here is to make sure your baby is fully asleep before transferring them. If they have literally just dropped off, they are likely to startle as soon as you begin to lower them. You can test this by putting your finger on their palm and seeing if they grip it. In theory, if they are fully asleep their hand will be relaxed and they won't grip. If you can wait ten minutes or so after they fall asleep this is optimum.

2. Lower your baby (very slowly!) into the cot on their side. Your baby's startle reflex (the Moro reflex) is activated when we lower babies on to their back (in theory, this should have faded by this age, but they can still retain the feeling of falling backwards). Make sure their bottom touches the cot first, then the rest of their body – this minimises this natural reflex. Once they are in, gently roll them on to their back (for safe sleeping).

3. Keep a hand on their chest or tummy (or one hand on each!), with a very gentle pressure. We want to maintain physical contact with them so that it's not a shock and they don't realise they have been moved.

4. Very gently and slowly, remove the pressure of your hand, until you can remove it entirely and then you can creep out!

5. Your baby may stay asleep for a few hours or they may only stay asleep for a short time. If it's the latter, you may want to consider some of the following methods to help lengthen that sleep.

## DREAM FEEDS

A dream feed is when parents rouse their baby and feed them late at night, just before they go to bed. Most parents I have worked with over the years do this at around 10.30/11pm. The idea is to manipulate your baby's longest stretch of sleep to be after this feed. For smaller babies, you might get all the way to 3am for the next feed. If you are bottle-feeding (formula or expressed breast milk) your partner might like to give the dream feed, so you get a longer chunk of sleep. If your baby is a bit older, a dream feed could be all you need for them to make it all the way through to morning. Some babies will fully wake if you go to do this, while others might stay asleep while you give the feed. It doesn't really matter – there are no set rules. Some families will fully wake and change a nappy; you can do whatever works. Dream feeds don't work for everyone, so it is all about experimenting and doing it if it feels right for your family.

## FADE IT OUT

Otherwise known as 'bedtime fading', this is a super slow, gentle method that can be really effective, if you accept you could be in it for the long haul. Having said this, sometimes small changes over a week or two can have a fast impact when doing this. This approach will suit you if you feel worried about your baby crying or that you won't be able to respond quickly to your baby. It is important to note that, even with this method, I can't guarantee that your baby won't cry, but you will be with them every step of the way.

With this approach, we add something else in to help us 'fade' out the thing we want to change. For example, if you rock your baby to sleep and want to move away from that, you could rock to sleep and also pat your baby's bottom. As each night goes on, you begin to rock less, but continue to pat. This way your baby gets used to a new way of falling asleep, which you can then eventually fade out too! We want to make sure that the new thing is preferable to or easier to move away from the original thing we are fading out.

An example of this approach:

- **Night 1:** Rock to sleep as usual.
- **Night 2:** Rock to sleep and pat your baby's bum at the same time.

- **Night 3:** Rock intermittently and pat your baby's bum at the same time.
- **Night 4:** Rock a little bit, then stay still and pat your baby's bum.
- **Night 5:** No rocking, just hold and pat your baby's bum.
- **Night 6:** Hold to sleep with some intermittent patting of the bum.
- **Night 7:** Hold to sleep with no patting.
- **Night 8:** Put down in their cot almost asleep after some holding.
- **Night 9:** Put down awake and (hopefully) you won't need to pat or rock anymore!

One of the common challenges with fade it out is fading out feeding to sleep, especially with breastfeeding (although *lots* of babies also fall asleep on their bottle).

It might look like this:

- **Night 1:** Feed to sleep as usual.
- **Night 2:** Feed to sleep and gently pat your baby's bum at the same time (you could exchange patting for swaying, singing or sssh-ing).
- **Night 3:** Feed until just before baby falls asleep while patting their bum. If they cry, then re-latch them, and pat their bum again. This is just about practising.
- **Night 4:** Feed them as usual, with some patting, and try unlatching them before they fall asleep – try replacing the nipple with the pad of your finger with a firm pressure against their mouth (see tip below). This can sometimes be enough for them to relax.
- **Night 5:** Feed until they slow down and are falling asleep. Unlatch them and pat them gently in your arms. You can now try putting them down into their sleep space awake or a little sleepy.

- **Night 6:** Put them down wide awake in their sleep space after their feed. You can continue to pat (or other sleep association) until they are calm. If they are calm, you should try to leave the room. If they begin to cry at any point during this process, you can pause for a moment, or pick them straight up and latch them back on.
- **Night 7:** If you have got to this point, you might want to continue doing this if it is working for you – or you could move on to one of the other methods detailed in the book.

Some people find it useful to change the location of the feed, or change where it sits in the bedtime routine. Doing the feed in your front room can help keep them awake at the breast or bottle. Although dimmed lights help us to sleep, in this instance we are trying to keep them awake, so it's okay for this to be in a well-lit room. You can try doing the feed before their bath, but I generally don't recommend this – feeding before sleep can help facilitate sleep, as breast milk contains sleep-inducing hormones, and feeding from a bottle is also relaxing for baby. I tend to advise feeding out of their sleeping bag and then putting them into it after the bedtime feed, as one of the steps of their bedtime routine.

> A little tip here: if your baby feeds to sleep either on the breast or bottle, try unlatching them and then putting your finger across their lips. Do this very quickly! The pressure of your finger can sometimes be enough to keep them settled.

You might also look at fading out a sleep behaviour just on its own, without adding in something else. For example, you might bounce your baby to sleep on a birthing ball (I have seen this many times during my practice). To 'fade' this out, you might follow the steps below:

- **Night 1:** Bounce as usual, but stop intermittently, taking time to pause with some stillness.
- **Night 2:** Bounce occasionally, until baby calms, and then have some stillness.
- **Night 3:** Sit on the ball and hold baby. If baby gets upset, bounce a little. Have longer periods of stillness.
- **Night 4:** Try holding to sleep.
- **Night 5:** Attempt to put baby down in their sleep space.

The idea is that this way you slowly get baby accustomed to falling asleep without being bounced.

This fade it out method still follows the idea that, in order to see change, we need to make change, but the change happens very gradually. I have used 'Night 1', 'Night 2' and so forth here to demonstrate that these steps should take place on successive nights. However, you may find that you're not ready to move on to the next step the very next night – in some cases it could take weeks or even months.

This is a great method if you are worried about not responding to your baby quickly. It is entirely responsive and gentle. Some families are not comfortable with any level of crying, but we can't stop our babies crying altogether and they are likely to communicate to us when something is changing. This method is suitable for all babies, but it's especially great for those with a more sensitive nature.

The drawback is that it can feel painfully slow if you are in the midst of a sleep crisis and need rapid change for your family. You need to be prepared that it can take some weeks or months to see any progress. You might start with this method and then graduate to one of the other methods below.

## CAMPING OUT

Otherwise known as accompanied or assisted crying (and many other names and interpretations!), with this approach, you essentially stay with your baby in their room. This is often on a chair or sitting next to the cot or crib, or it could be on a mattress, so you are sleeping on the floor next to them. You comfort your baby whenever they need it, but the idea is that they stay in their own sleep space and you don't get them out. This means that you are comforting your baby while they are in their cot, whether that's patting, rubbing or shushing. You could stay with them until they drop off or you might try to leave just before they do. I tend to advise leaving just before they fall asleep, so that they get used to doing this on their own. That might be something you work towards very slowly.

Each time your baby wakes in the night, you reassure them and, gradually, as they learn to settle themselves, you can have less input. If your baby is waking really frequently, you can just stay next to them rather than coming in and out of the room. This is a slower method but it can feel easier for some families to just remain in the room than dashing in and out if you are feeling stressed.

This method can take a while depending on your baby, and you'll need to keep challenging boundaries to progress. Some families simply get stuck comforting by the cot and find it hard to move on from there. Continuing to change how you do things is key with this method – remember to keep working your way up the staircase (see page 169).

As with all of these methods, camping out needs to be tailored to the baby and family in question. As a parent you need to really tune into your baby and how they are reacting. Working out whether they need you or not can be a tricky one.

Camping out might look like this:

- Night 1: you put baby down awake in their cot (or drowsy if going slower). If your baby is calm, you move towards the door. If they cry, you sit or lie with them (either on a chair or mattress). You continue to comfort them every time they cry. This might look like placing a hand on them and sshing, or patting, or singing – whatever works for your baby and offers reassurance that you are there. Some people repeat their sleepy phrase (see page 164).
- Night 2: more of the same, but hopefully they are a little calmer.
- Night 3: you might try to leave before they actually nod off.
- Nights 4–14: hopefully, within the space of two weeks or so, they will be calm enough for you to leave them to it!

Some parents find this is a good transition method when they are moving baby into their own room. The parent can sleep on a mattress next to the cot for a few nights, or even a few weeks while baby gets used to it. You could also sit on a chair – this leads into the next method.

It is also okay if you continue to stay with your child indefinitely until they fall asleep. It might be that you feel comfortable with this boundary and that your child gets a settled night's sleep. You might decide you have reached the place you wanted to get to and you are happy staying here. Some parents continue this for several years.

### *Going it alone*

*I met a single mum and her baby, Mateo. Mateo was 11 months old at the time. Mum had been co-sleeping with Mateo since he turned four months old and his sleep had really gone haywire. She found that she got a little more sleep if they slept in the same bed – it meant she was able to comfort him next to her, rather than keep getting up. It also meant if he wanted to breastfeed, she could just roll over and feed him, and then roll back again.*

*The reason she had got in touch was she felt like it was time for him to sleep in his own sleep space, and that she wanted to get a more settled night. She said that at 11 months, it was time for her to use her own duvet as it was designed – to actually get under it! (She had been pushing it to the side of the bed behind her for safe sleeping, so it didn't touch Mateo.)*

*We spoke at length about his personality and how she felt about sleep. We decided that she would stay in the room to settle him, but he would be in his own room, at last (her words!). It felt bittersweet she said – her little best friend and bed companion had been such a comfort to her too, but she knew they would both get the rest they needed if he moved into his own space. She had a cot set up, in a beautiful nursery – she had curated that room with the utmost love and attention. We also moved a single mattress onto the floor next to his cot. We put him down into his cot wide awake at bedtime, and she said good night but lay down on the mattress. Initially he thought it was a game. He was crawling around and pulling himself up. He was definitely tired at this point (we made sure his routine was spot on). He then started getting upset. Mum sat up and put her hand through the bars and patted his mattress. She put her hands on his side (he was lying on his side) and said, 'Night night Mateo, sleep now' (this was their sleepy phrase). He cried on and off for about ten minutes. He calmed and fell asleep holding her hand in the end. She was able to roll over and go to sleep on the single mattress on the floor.*

*Mateo still woke three times during the night and each time Mum did the same thing (the first waking he was awake for six minutes, the second was two minutes and the third was twenty minutes, but he did go back to sleep). Across the following two weeks the night wakings reduced to just one, and he was going to sleep very quickly. Mum was able to be completely hands-off, but just say her sleepy phrase so he could hear it. On the fifteenth night she said good night to him and moved back to her own bed. She said she heard him on the monitor, he stirred and wriggled and got himself back to sleep. He slept through until 6am, which was an absolute result for her. She was an early bird and didn't mind a fairly early start. It turns out that Mateo wakes around 6am to this day – he's just wired that way.*

## THE DISAPPEARING CHAIR
## (THE CHAIR METHOD)

This is essentially the same as the camping out method, but you specifically use a chair. It starts next to the cot and, depending on how quickly you progress, over the coming days or weeks each night it moves a little further away from baby until you are out of the room. I tend to find that this method works better for older babies who are more aware of your presence in the room. Again, the idea is that you are not getting them out of their cot, but you will be giving verbal reassurance from the chair (your sleepy phrase or 'sssh sssh', for example).

This method can feel quite empowering in some ways as you have a clear rule: 'I am sitting on this chair until you fall asleep.' For parents who find all the rules and timings of other methods confusing, it can be a simple way to approach sleep changes.

This method can be ineffective with babies at the younger end of the age spectrum as they don't have much awareness of the chair itself and where it is in the room, and so can become frustrated and get upset wondering why you are just sitting there and not doing anything. Also, if you have the room very dark, they can't see you anyway.

If this is the case for you and your baby, I am a firm believer that you should be able to go and comfort your baby with a hand on them or even pick them up if you want to (see next method below). Each method must have some flexibility for you to react in the moment.

It might look like this:

- **Night 1:** you put your baby down awake in their cot (or drowsy if going slower). If your baby is calm, you sit on a chair next to the cot. If they cry, continue to sit with them. You can either choose to reassure them verbally (with your sleepy phrase) and stay on the chair, or you can put your hands into the cot to comfort them – whatever works to give them reassurance that you are there.
- **Night 2:** more of the same, but hopefully they are a little calmer.
- **Night 3:** you try to move the chair away from the cot by a couple of feet.
- **Nights 4–14:** each night you move the chair further and further away, towards the door, until you are out of the room and baby can fall asleep independently.

## PICK UP TO COMFORT

Although this is not a method that I use very often, picking up your baby to comfort them is never wrong. You must trust your intuition and do what feels right for you.

For this method, you put your baby down awake and, each time they get upset, you pick them up to comfort them. In theory, once they are calm you put them down. However, in practice they may well still be upset or protest as soon as you put them down. The idea is that you repeat this until baby finally gives up and settles themselves to sleep.

I think this method can be confusing for babies as it sends mixed messages and, in my experience, many babies find it over-stimulating and it can actually obstruct them falling asleep. You need to be prepared that, for some babies, this method could extend how long it takes for them to fall asleep at bedtime. Having said that, for some families, if they get baby's level of tiredness right and they are really ready for sleep, it can work.

It can feel momentarily kinder than some of the following methods as you physically comfort/cuddle your little one. However, it's short-lived as you will need to put them down again (when baby will likely cry even harder!). Babies with a more sensitive temperament might find it too distressing each time you put them back down, and it can feel distressing and confusing for parents too. Your baby might be arching their back and screaming in your arms as you wrestle them, which is not very calming for sleep!

## CONTROLLED CRYING

Otherwise known as the interval method, interval crying, the Ferber method, graduated extinction, controlled comforting, quick checks or graduated crying, this method can be very hard as it involves putting your baby down awake and allowing them to cry for intervals of time before returning to comfort them. The idea is that you don't lift them out of their sleep space, but rather comfort them by patting, sshing, stroking or with verbal reassurance. With some versions of this, the intervals of time will increase after each check in, and there are others where the interval of time always stays the same.

If this method is done in an empowering way, allowing parents to tune into and interpret their baby's cries, it can be a very effective way to help your baby adjust to a different way of falling asleep. This method is probably the one that has the most alternative names and adaptations. I also believe that this is generally the most popular method in the evidence and literature that we have around this subject. The reason being is that it does work – for *most* babies.

It is important to be prepared that controlled crying can feel distressing for both parent and baby. Especially if bedtime isn't timed right, baby could be crying for a long time. For those who are uncomfortable with any unattended crying, this isn't a good choice. It is really important that with this method you get your timings right – do not try to put baby to bed before they are ready. You need sleep pressure (see page 29) on your side. Babies are far more likely to accept a new way of falling asleep at bedtime rather than any other time during the day, or even later on in the night.

Trying this approach might look something like this:

- **Step 1:** Put baby down awake or drowsy in their cot and leave the room. If they start to cry, set a timer for two minutes (this is just an example – the time could be shorter or longer). If it gets to two minutes and your baby is still crying, you go in and reassure them with your sleepy phrase and a pat, sssh, stroke, kiss or whatever your baby tends to like. Then you leave again for another two minutes, and then you return – *if* they are still crying – to comfort. You repeat this process until they fall asleep. If your baby is calm or not crying, you don't need to go in.
- **Step 2:** You continue this process for every wake-up during the night.
- **Step 3:** For the ongoing nights, some people will extend the time that they are out of the room – two minutes, then three minutes, then four minutes, and so on. This can sometimes feel confusing and arbitrary, so do what makes sense to you. You can keep your time limit the same, or extend it, or even shorten it!

I like to react to the baby in the moment – if it feels like they are getting distressed, you could go in sooner than your allotted time, or you could leave it longer if it sounds like they are calming. I think it is important to be flexible and to be able to change tack in the moment if you need to. For some laid-back babies this method can work in a few nights; for others it really doesn't suit them and it is better to start off more gradually with one of the other methods outlined earlier in this chapter. If this method doesn't fit with your parenting ethos, definitely choose another approach.

## THE CRY IT OUT METHOD

This method literally means letting baby cry out until they tire and fall asleep. With this method, you put baby down awake, walk away and don't return until the morning. You don't comfort the baby or check in on them (other than using a monitor if you have one). It is entirely unresponsive, and it is what it says on the tin – letting them cry it out. It feels unnecessary when we have other methods we can choose from. I believe we need to have the flexibility to be able to check in on and reassure our babies, which this method doesn't provide.

It can also feel traumatic, especially if we can't be certain that we have covered all other bases – if you can't be 100 per cent sure baby is well, or that you have hit their sweet spot for bedtime for example. If your baby wasn't ready for bed it could result in a lot of crying, which would be totally unfair on everyone.

# WHEN YOUR CHOSEN METHOD ISN'T WORKING

It's important to be flexible with whatever method you choose. If you try it and decide it's not working for your baby, you can absolutely stop, take a step back and reassess. However, if you are trying something new it is important to give it a good shot. Some parents give up quickly, saying things haven't worked, when in fact they just needed a bit more time on it.

It is worth noting that you might find the method you choose to be far easier at the beginning of the night than in the early hours. This is because of our old friend sleep pressure. It is much higher at the beginning of the night and almost non-existent by the morning. This means that your baby is far more likely to accept a new way of falling asleep before midnight. After that, I find that, as each hour goes on, they can find it trickier to get back to sleep.

It isn't uncommon to use one method at the beginning of the night and revert to something else in the early hours. There isn't anything wrong with this, but some parents get a bit stuck this way. If you want drastic change, you need to stick to one thing all night. For example, if you bring baby into your bed halfway through the night, it might work well for you in that moment. However, it might mean that you set a precedent and then baby begins to expect this, and essentially just waits for you to take them out. It's all a learning journey to see what works for you and your family, but I want to point this out so that you understand why something might feel like it is working one minute, and not the next!

If it feels like your plan generally isn't working for you or your baby, ask yourself the following questions:

- *Have I given it enough time?* I have seen it many times when parents give up after one attempt. Give it a few attempts, a few days or even a few weeks before you give up. Remember, changing both our baby's habits and our own takes time.

- *Am I being consistent in my approach?* While you can always change your mind, perhaps you are responding differently to your little one each time. Giving a clear message feels fairer to everyone.
- *Is my little one tired enough for sleep or am I trying to force it?* Sometimes moving bedtime or naptime a little later can help your little one to accept a new way of falling asleep. And, of course, if we are attempting a nap or bedtime too soon, before their sleep pressure is high enough, we will have a battle on our hands.
- *Is their bedtime too late?* On the flip side, sometimes a fractious baby who has been awake for too long can be hard to calm down (remember what I said about keeping calm?).
- *Is there something else going on?* Is your little one in physical discomfort? Is something bothering them? Are they unwell? It is always worth checking with your doctor if you are unsure.
- *Have I chosen the right method for my little one?* Perhaps your little one is hardier than you thought and they would respond better with a faster change. Or perhaps your little one is more sensitive, in which case pick something more gradual.
- *Are my own experiences and triggers holding me back from making change?* None of us likes to hear crying. Take a step back and ask yourself if your little one's cry is actually a cry of distress or does it sound like they are falling asleep? If we rush in too quickly, we can sometimes get in the way. Challenging our own beliefs about crying can be the key (see page 39).

---

It's all a learning journey to see what works
for you and your family.

---

## SLEEP TRAINING AN OLDER BABY

It is never too late to work on improving sleep. You might find that an older baby (eight to twelve months old) is more mobile and likely to sit up or stand up when you put them into their sleep space and you are changing the way you get them to sleep. You can still use any of the methods that I have detailed in this chapter, but be prepared for them to sit or stand. Don't push or force them to lie or sit down – they need to do it of their own accord. Don't turn it into a game or a battle. You can gently encourage them by patting the mattress or lying down next to them. They will eventually sit and lie down themselves.

## *Sleep crisis*

*I worked with a baby called Willow, who was six months old. Her parents were, literally, at breaking point. Her mum had emailed me at 2am, saying she was in floods of tears and she couldn't do it anymore. She hadn't slept for more than an hour and a half in one go for six months. The parents' relationship was strained, they had no time together and she was started to resent becoming a mother. I arrived at their home late morning to a very sad-looking mum and a concerned-looking dad. I asked how much Willow had slept that morning and they told me it was 40 minutes at 8.45am. I knew that this meant she would be ready for her lunchtime nap by around 12ish. We talked through absolutely everything – from pregnancy, birth and every month after. They talked to me about how they settled her (either with a feed, rocking or even driving her around in the car at night!). This couple were in what I would call a 'sleep crisis'.*

*We talked about the sleep methods, and I knew they needed some quick change. In spite of how broken her parents were, Willow was a cheerful little baby. She seemed unfazed by my presence in her home. They had just started weaning so she had a little food, and then we decided to try her nap in her cot (she was normally driven around). We introduced a pre-nap wind down – a little story from Mum, a cuddle and a lullaby, and then into her sleeping bag. We put Willow down, wide awake, into her cot. This was at 12.20pm, as Willow had managed the morning really well. Mum and Dad said good night and tried leaving the room. Initially Willow was just blowing raspberries, but then she began to cry. We had decided they would try controlled crying, see how they got on and consider changing if they felt uncomfortable.*

*Willow cried for two minutes and her dad entered the room. He put his hands on her chest and said 'Sssh, it's okay, I'm here, night night' and walked out again. She cried again, for two minutes. They were about to go in and I told them to stop – there was a pause in her crying. It suddenly reduced. I told them to wait for another minute. She started again, so Dad went in to do the same reassurance. When he left, she let out a big cry, and suddenly went quiet. She turned over and went to sleep. They were floored. It was the first time she had ever got herself to sleep. She woke after 40 minutes and we tried the same, but she showed no signs of calming. They got her up and carried on with their day – I suggested they all get out for a nice walk and fresh air. I also suggested a longer third nap to catch up, and to do this on the move as usual to avoid any more upset. They were to start the method again at bedtime. Now this was the real game changer. Willow cried for three minutes and went to sleep. She then slept for six hours straight, woke for a feed and then slept until 6.30am. That was the day their life changed.*

## REFRAMING YOUR LANGUAGE

Language 'reframing' is a common coaching tool, which can be so useful when working with clients, but also for parents to have in mind when they are looking at sleep, for a bit of self-coaching. I am a big fan of reframing our language.

Here are some common examples that I hear from parents when they embark on a sleep plan:

- *She refuses to sleep in her cot!* I like to reframe this as 'She is not used to sleeping in her cot.'
- *He started crying immediately!* I like to reframe this as 'He is communicating to me that something is different.'
- *Why are we doing this? It's a nightmare!* I like to reframe this as 'We have made this decision to work on our little one's sleep to get the rest we need. The process feels hard, because it is hard.'
- *This is never going to work!* I like to reframe this as 'I am giving myself and my baby the space to make gradual changes in how we approach sleep. It will take as long as it takes.'
- *I am never going to sleep again!* I like to reframe this as 'There will always be sleep on the horizon. The sun will continue to come up and go down, and one day my baby will sleep through the night, even if we choose to do nothing right now, or if we try again tomorrow.'
- *What if this doesn't work?* I like to reframe this as 'What would it mean to my baby and our family if this were to work?'
- *I am trying to force a routine when my baby doesn't want one.* I like to reframe this as 'I am setting up the best foundations for my baby to have a predictable, but flexible bedtime. We have chosen to let go of the chaos and embrace regularity. My baby is happy if I am happy.'

- *I can't handle my baby's crying!* I like to reframe this as 'Crying is a normal part of babyhood and I never have to leave my baby unattended if it doesn't feel right for me.'

You get the gist! It can be hard not to get bogged down by negative thought patterns and beliefs. Ultimately, you call the shots. If you want to do this, you can. It doesn't mean that it will be a straight road (it will probably be pretty bendy), but you will be continuing on a path towards the settled night's sleep that you deserve.

## SOMETHING FOR EVERYONE

All of the methods I have described in this chapter are valid. I believe there is something here for everyone. It is important for me to demystify these methods and to show up with practical solutions. Unfortunately, none of these are a magic pill to transform your little one's sleep overnight, but that doesn't mean that by trying things out, you won't see rapid change.

---

Whatever your culture, beliefs or physical set-up,
you can work on sleep if you want to.

---

Some families I have worked with have seen very quick change using the methods above. Sometimes it's just about working out what the missing part of the puzzle is for your baby. It might be how they settle, but it could just as easily be a good balance of day and night sleep or something in their sleep environment that is a barrier to sleep. It could be a medical concern or something else. It is our job to remain curious and non-judgemental. We shouldn't judge others for their parenting choices, or ourselves. It is not cruel or damaging to use controlled crying with your baby, nor is it spoiling your baby if you share a bed with them. I would encourage you to remain open-minded about your little one's sleep, and don't knock a method until you've tried it.

I hope that with all the information you have read so far, you feel really prepared for your sleep journey with your little one, whatever that may look like, armed with all the knowledge on how to improve sleep, how to work on it if you want to and how to set up a great environment for your baby to sleep in.

The next part of this book is going to cover all of the other things that can happen with sleep, to prepare you and help you protect against any challenges you might face.

## KEY TAKEAWAYS

**1.** Understand what is going on with your baby's sleep.

**2.** Understand how to identify your window of opportunity.

**3.** Set your baby up for success.

**4.** There is an approach for everyone – choose the method that is right for you and change it if you need to.

**5.** Get the settled night that you need.

# PART 4

# 9

# FUTURE-PROOFING YOUR BABY'S SLEEP

Even if you have managed to make changes to your baby's sleep and are getting a good night's sleep yourself, you may well still face challenges along the way. I want you to be well-equipped to face potential bumps in the road and give you some solid advice on how to be fully prepared for these.

## INTRODUCING ANOTHER CAREGIVER

It is common for babies to prefer one parent or caregiver in particular. This makes sense because it is how they survive – if any old stranger could pick them up and settle them, they wouldn't survive very long in 'the wild' (back in prehistoric times, for example!). But it doesn't make it any less frustrating when you (if you are the preferred parent) want or need a break. It might be that you want to go out for the evening, or you are working, or you just want to share the load. It can also be frustrating for the non-preferred parent or carer when they want to get involved too.

Your baby may have become used to one person caring for them at bedtime. So, if you are the one who always settles your baby in a particular way, they will be surprised when someone else tries to do it, probably in a different style to what they are used to.

> We need to give our babies credit – they are smart
> enough to realise it's another person who smells
> different, sounds different and does things differently.

In Chapter 11, I talk more about the dynamics of your relationship when it comes to sleep and sharing the care, but for now here are some tips on how you can introduce another caregiver at sleep times – be it your partner or a grandparent, cousin, auntie, uncle, friend or babysitter.

1. If you are introducing someone, do it slowly – you can start by just having them in the general area during the bedtime routine. Hovering in the background and talking to you and your baby is good.

2. Each night try getting them a little bit more involved – for example, let them take over during the bath, or they could lift the baby out and pass them to you, or dry baby and get them dressed with you present, and you can gradually try leaving or being less involved.

3. Even if you are breastfeeding, you can still pass baby to their other caregiver to settle them. It can be hard if they are used to settling with the boob or if you do something in particular (like they play with your hair or you cuddle them in a certain way), but I promise they will still settle for someone else.

4. Giving the caregiver time to find their own style is key – they won't do things exactly how you do them, and babies are clever, they learn that different people do things differently.

5. Have a conversation beforehand so everyone knows what the plan is. Explain your bedtime boundaries and agree on a plan together.

6. Stay safe in the knowledge that your baby will eventually fall asleep with someone else, as hard as this can be. I have never

known a baby stay awake the entire night. Try to relax and trust in the process.

In case you don't have the luxury of a slow introduction (perhaps you have to introduce a new caregiver at bedtime in an emergency), it helps to have your baby's approximate routine and their likes and dislikes written down somewhere.

## WORKING TOGETHER

When you implement a sleep-training method, it is fine for both parents (and any other caregivers who might look after your baby in the evening) to be involved. It is also okay if just one parent is responsible. It's about doing whatever works for your family, and who is available. You may find that your baby might respond better initially to one parent.

It can help to have moral support while you are making changes, and to share the load if you are dealing with night waking.

What's most important when there is more than one person involved in trying to implement a sleep change is that you are all on the same page and using the same method.

## TRAVELLING WITH YOUR BABY

Many parents worry that travelling with their baby will 'mess up' the sleep work they have done because of deviating from the norm and not being able to strictly stick to their routine. I always advise that if you can stick to your usual sleep routine and it is not stressful to do so, then do it. If you can't, then let it go and don't stress. On the day of travel it often all goes out of the window anyway, so you can either be mindful of timings when you start your holiday or just fly by the seat of your pants.

Here are my top tips for managing your baby's sleep on holiday:

1. Hire a reputable babysitter if you plan to leave your baby for an evening – you could request to meet them beforehand, so you feel comfortable.

2. If possible, stay in a villa rather than a hotel so you can put baby to bed as normal and eat in the next room using a monitor or have your baby in the room with you in a travel cot if they are younger.

3. If you are sharing a room with your baby when you don't normally, use white noise (see page 68), if possible, to minimise disturbance, and stay quiet and still while baby is getting to sleep. Once they are asleep, most won't be disrupted while you are moving around in the evening. They tend to be more sensitive in the early hours of the morning (so be quiet if you get up to go for a wee!).

   In my time, I have moved furniture around in hotel rooms and put travel cots in different corners of the room to see what works! Some hotel rooms have dividers or a sliding screen, which can be great if your baby is easily stimulated by your presence.

4. Do the bedtime routine as normal, but put your baby to bed in their buggy and walk to a restaurant/bar and hope that they sleep! You can then transfer them once you are back (see page 171 for transfer tips). You could also have baby sleep in a sling (make sure you are following safe baby-wearing guidance – see page 71). Don't worry if you need to give an extra 'bedtime' feed if your baby wakes up on your return. Just go with it.

5. Give them a longer or later naptime and keep them up with you over dinner. This might mean a second meal for them or entertaining them with toys.

6. Take a buggy that can lie flat so that, if you are doing naps on the go (hopefully round a dreamy swimming pool or beach), your baby will be able to drift off comfortably. Try to keep your little one in the shade or use a parasol for the buggy. Make sure you monitor their temperature and never cover the buggy with a muslin, towel or blanket – this makes it heat up like a greenhouse. There are some designed-for-purpose sunshades on the market now – make sure you choose one that is safety-tested.

I generally find that little ones who are used to getting themselves to sleep are very adaptable when you travel. They will surprise you. And for those who are more sensitive or who are not sleeping independently, it is okay to do more than you usually would to settle them. This might mean bed-sharing when you don't normally do it. If that is you, don't worry about it – just make sure you follow the safety guidelines (see page 53).

> Wherever you are going, take your little one's favourite comforter (see page 155) or some familiar toys and your baby's slept-in sheet. This is helpful when you arrive at your destination to make their cot or room feel more like home (bear in mind safe sleep guidance around toys – see page 51).

### Travelling by plane

If you are flying, I highly recommend taking a baby sling/carrier. This means that you can carry your baby with your hands free and potentially rock or sway them to sleep on the plane. It is also useful when you are boarding the plane and have lots of bits to carry! I have spent many flights over the years walking up and down and jiggling my babies in the aisle. It also means that if they do drop off you can eat, drink or read a book. Don't forget to take a change of clothes for baby, and you! I have had many a spillage – and vomit – on me (it's also handy to have spare clothes if your bags were ever to get lost).

You can check with your airline in advance whether they have a bassinet available – this often depends on how many babies they have on the flight. If you have the option to reserve one, I highly recommend doing so. It is more expensive, but you could reserve your baby their own seat on the plane. I have seen some airlines now allowing seat extenders (which you can buy) which unfold to make a space for your baby to lie down in. Do check with the airline, and of course make sure it is set up according to the manufacturer's guidelines so that it is safe.

## JET LAG

This is a biggie that I have been asked about so many times over the years. Here are my tips:

1. Exposure to natural light really influences our internal body clocks. When you get to your destination, try to get outside in the light as it will help you and your baby adapt to the local time at your destination.
2. Movement is great to tire us out, but also to tell our bodies that it's daytime, especially if you have a toddler or baby on the move. Burning off some energy in the airport before departure can also be useful!
3. Eat at the local time. When we eat also has a big impact on our internal body clocks. Try to eat during

daylight hours. If your baby wakes particularly hungry, don't be afraid to feed them though – don't withhold feeds.

4.  Depending on how far you are travelling, you might want to stick to your normal schedule. For example, if you were to go to Europe from the UK you might just adjust your daytime schedule to 8am to 8pm for example (obviously time differences vary).

5.  If it's a longer distance and you want to start adjusting before you go, you can treat it like a clock change. So, you can prepare your baby in advance by moving their bedtime and entire schedule in 15-minute increments to be closer to the local time at your destination before you leave (or even when you arrive). This can make a big time difference less of a shock to the system. If you can turn a five-hour difference into a three- to four-hour difference, it will make the transition quicker.

6.  Make sure you have plenty of snacks if your baby eats solids. If they sleep through a meal, they could wake up hungry (and you could do the same! Don't forget to take care of yourself too).

7.  I tend to find that babies adapt quicker than adults as they nap during the day and can catch up on lost sleep. However, don't let them 'over nap' otherwise you might end up with a very wakeful baby at night. If this does happen, try to keep things dark, quiet and boring during the night-time.

8.  Remember, if it all goes out of the window, just roll with it. You will all adapt eventually.

I have always tried to plan train or plane journeys for when my children are going to be taking their longest nap. This isn't always possible, but bear it in mind if you have options.

## GETTING OUT AND ABOUT WITH YOUR BABY

A common concern for parents is getting out and 'having a life' while protecting their little one's sleep routine. This could be social occasions, or it could be a weekly baby class, or just you wanting to get out and see your friends. Having a baby who sleeps well should not mean you are under lock and key, and I think it's vital that you have a social life. It might look different to your social life pre-children, but we still need to socialise. It is good for us, and for our babies.

Don't ever let anyone tell you that you must stay at home all day, every day for your baby to sleep well. It's a common misconception about sleep training and sleep work in general.

While it's handy if your baby can have naps in their cot (and for some families it's the Holy Grail they are aiming for), it shouldn't get in the way of you having a life.

Here are my tips for getting out and about during the day:

1. Some babies struggle to have long naps while on the go. You might try absolutely everything and they just won't go down for more than 30–45 minutes. If this is the case, often it is worth leaning into it, letting it go and accepting it.

2. You can try to time the naps so you are on the move. If your little one needs a nap, make sure you are walking them in the pram/sling or driving in the car at the time. Be mindful that you are moving again at around the 30–45-minute mark. This will hopefully help them to link sleep cycles (see page 30).

3. You could try using a portable white noise machine and a cover for your buggy. Be mindful not to use a blanket or muslin – you should only use something safety-tested and designed for purpose.

4. You could think about reorganising your day if you know you are going out. For example, you might give your little one a longer nap than usual (if they will do it!) before you leave, and then push through to an early bedtime or a short nap later. It's worth playing around with their routine and not stressing out if there's a day when naps don't go to the usual plan.

5. Make sure baby is dressed in easy layers so you can either remove them or cover baby up depending on the temperature. We don't want baby to overheat if we go from outside to inside, so always aim to remove hats and coats. Always remove rain covers when you go inside so that baby doesn't get too hot.

6. If it's a regular baby class, pick wisely. I have dodged many lunchtime classes in my time – I think sometimes it's not worth it if you are going to have a tired, miserable baby on your hands, but then again it depends on your baby. Some are more laid back and flexible than others who need their nap at the same time each day.

7. I'm often asked about weddings and evening events. I would do the same as on holiday – aim to do a mini bedtime routine, and put them to bed in their buggy, to transfer them to their cot later. Or give them a later, longer nap and keep them up for the evening with you. It's often trial and error, and hopefully you'll have some willing helpers in friends and family to support you.

> Sometimes travelling later in the day can mean a 'danger nap' – this is when your little one sleeps too long or too close to bedtime. If this can't be avoided, don't worry – just push their bedtime a little later than usual.

## SLEEP AND SICKNESS

During a child's early years (especially during the winter months), it can feel like snotty noses go on forever. It is normal for sleep to be disrupted or for a child to struggle to settle when they don't feel well, but it can be frustrating if you feel like every time you get into a good sleep routine another illness pops up. Try not to worry and keep in mind that every stage is just a phase. If the illness isn't obvious, but you feel like something is wrong, always seek advice from your doctor or emergency medical support if necessary.

A parent's intuition is strong and you know your baby – if you feel like something is up, it probably is.

So, what can you do to help your baby?

**1.** Bear in mind supplementation as a first line of defence. If your little one is having less than 500ml of formula per day, they need a vitamin D supplement. Vitamin D helps our immune systems and a lack of it has been linked to sleep disruption. NHS guidance is that breastfed babies need a vitamin D supplement from birth, regardless of whether you are taking one yourself. Getting outside in the fresh air and sleeping well are also really helpful for our health in general, and our baby's health. Besides vitamin D, children up to age five should also be supplemented with vitamins A and C (again, providing they are having less than 500ml of formula a day).

2. When we are poorly, the body needs to rest – sleep literally heals. Your little one might need extra naps in the day or may in fact sleep less due to being uncomfortable – they might have a fever, a cough or potentially be congested if they have a cold. Factoring in some rest time to your days can help. My rules around the TV go out of the window when an illness is in the home (normally we should try to keep TV to a minimum for babies).

3. Your baby might need extra feeds or fluids. If our noses are blocked, we tend to wake up feeling thirsty as we breathe through our mouths. Also, if they have been sweating from a fever, they will be more thirsty than usual. Don't worry about giving extra feeds – you won't go backwards with sleep. Keep an eye on the number of wet and dirty nappies your baby produces. If you are ever concerned, always speak to your doctor.

4. Your little one may want more contact with you at night than usual, so it is always okay to give that extra reassurance or cuddles. Make sure you have some support in place wherever possible during the day (or night) so you can rest – we spend so much energy looking after our little ones that we often forget about ourselves.

5. As you know by now, I am a fan of baby massage (see page 115). You can gently work on their chest to release congestion – imagine drawing angel wings across your baby's chest with your hands. You can also very gently work around the nose – use sweeping motions with your thumbs on either side of the nose and across the cheeks. This helps move snot down and out! I am very wary of 'snot suckers' on the market. It only takes one false move and you can damage a very sensitive little nostril, so I don't generally recommend these.

6. You can try a dehumidifier or a vapour plug-in in your baby's room. I am cautious with these too, though – always keep an eye on baby and note they are not suitable for babies under three months or pregnant women. I like to still have some air flow through the room when using these too. Vapour rubs should only be used on babies over six months old.

7. Make sure your little one is up to date with their vaccine schedule. These are at eight weeks, twelve weeks and sixteen weeks of age. Vaccines teach our immune systems how to protect our bodies from these dangerous diseases. They can literally save lives. You might find that your baby is unsettled after their vaccines, but this should be short-lived. You can give pain medication as advised by your doctor or practice nurse. They might sleep a lot more than usual or be a little fretful. As always, keep an eye on them and seek advice if you are concerned.

## SLEEP REGRESSIONS

There are things that can happen or influence sleep at any time, and are entirely individual, but are referred to by some as regressions at very specific stages and ages. But the only true sleep change – regression – is at around four months (although the change can happen anywhere between three and six months in my experience) – see Chapter 7.

I believe that the developmental changes, environmental influences and fluctuating health of your little one can cause 'blips' in their sleep but are not 'regressions'. When it comes to developmental changes, each child will roll over, crawl and walk at a different age – you can't pinpoint this to a certain week or month, so it certainly can't be tied to a change in sleep. There is no data to support the idea that changes in your little one's sleep are linked to any specific timeline.

When it comes to sleep changes, it is better to
observe your own baby and be curious
about their behaviour.

Be a detective, as outlined on page 116. I have known first hand of families dismissing fussy behaviour as a 'leap' or 'regression' when there has been something quite serious underlying, so if you have any concerns always contact your health visitor or GP.

Be reassured that sleep is not linear, and these 'blips' do just happen sometimes. In my professional and personal experience, the following things can influence sleep.

1. Moving home.
2. Starting nursery.
3. Going on holiday.
4. Illness.
5. The heat (very hot or cold weather).
6. Teething (although, in theory, this shouldn't cause too much disruption).
7. Learning to roll, crawl, stand, babble . . . !
8. Starting solids.
9. Allergies and reflux.
10. Nap transitions.

What you really want to know is how to handle these periods of disruption. The answer is the same as how to deal with sleep at any time – go back to basics:

- Look at your little one's health – is something bothering them? Do you need to see a doctor?
- Is there something in their sleep environment that is bothering them?

- Does their routine need tweaking (do they need a later bed-time or to drop a nap)?
- Have they been sleeping with you when poorly and just got used to it?
- Have they started solids too quickly?
- Is the weather very hot?
- Do they just need a bit more support than normal because there has been a big change?

The examples I could give are endless, but you get the picture. Be curious (see page 116), rule things out and then work on sleep environment, routine and how your baby settles.

## EARLY WAKING

I am afraid that most small people like to start the day early. It's a sad fact for many of us (especially us night owls!), but if we can adjust as parents and know that we are getting a decent night's sleep ahead of an early wake, it hopefully shouldn't be too painful. 'Early waking' is often the last piece of the puzzle when you are working on your little one's sleep. I have worked with many families over the years who have achieved a solid night's sleep, but their babies still wake up early. Later waking can be achieved with time, patience and a bit of trial and error. Keeping up with their ever-changing sleep needs is key and make sure those rooms are blacked out in the summer!

I consider anything earlier than 6am to be an 'early wake'. As far as I am concerned, it is pretty much night-time if it begins with a 5, whereas anything after 6am is fair game. You might be able to make some tweaks and push your baby's wake-up time a little later, but it really does depend on whether your baby is wired to be an early bird or not. Some children will be able to wake up at 7/7.30am, while with others you'll be lucky to see 6.30am. While there are plenty of things we can tweak and look at, sometimes we do have to relinquish our slow, late starts that we might have hoped for.

The things you *can* look at include:

1.  Is your baby's first nap of the day too early or too long? If this happens, it can serve to 'cement' their early wake. They can use their long nap to catch up on lost sleep at night and continue the cycle. Have a look at a 24-hour period and how long the night sleep is and how long the naps are. Can you tweak them so that sleep is taken in the early hours of the morning, rather than a long nap? Trying to stick to regular naptimes can also help.

2.  Have they simply slept enough overnight? This is where a later bedtime can help. I say later, but don't swing so far the other way that they are getting 'overtired' (see page 212), wired or upset.

3.  Is something in their environment disturbing them? Are they being woken by the birds, or your partner getting up, or something else? White noise can help here (see page 68). Is the sound of the heating coming on waking them? Are they waking cold? Rule out anything environmentally specific to your home and your set-up.

4.  Do they know how to get themselves back to sleep? If you helped them at the beginning of the night, they might simply be looking for you to return and do whatever it was you did before to help them. Remember, it's much easier to get to sleep at the beginning of the night (sleep pressure!) and much harder to get back to sleep in the early hours. Working on how your little one gets to sleep at night *might* be the key.

5.  If you have done absolutely everything you can and they are still waking early, a bit of surrender is good. By this I mean knowing that this is the time you get up and trying to get an

early night. Take it in turns with your partner to get up in the morning if possible, and factor some downtime into your day. A 15-minute nap after lunch (for you!) can do wonders to get you through the day. Don't nap for too long, though, or you won't be ready to go to bed early – remember, sleep pressure needs to be high enough for us to fall asleep and by napping we reduce that pressure. Naps are restorative and I highly recommend them, but just be mindful of how long you nap for.

## SPLIT NIGHTS

If your baby is waking up for hours in the middle of the night, we often refer to this as a 'split night'. This is not about baby waking and crying and trying to settle – this is when baby wants to get up and play, seems rested and shows no signs of going back to sleep. In my experience, there are a few common reasons for this:

1. Too much daytime sleep. We can easily fall into the trap of thinking what 'amazing' naps our babies are having, but, in fact, one person can only sleep so much in a 24-hour period. If your baby is taking long naps in the day, beyond an age-appropriate amount, this can cause wakefulness at night-time. It can be a tricky cycle to break, but tweaking naps during the day often solves it. You can also try a later bedtime potentially. Please note this doesn't apply to small babies – they need lots of daytime sleep to feel rested. For newborns it's more often that they have day and night confused – lots of natural light in the day and making sure they don't sleep through feeds during the day can help with this.

2. Going to bed too early. Perhaps they didn't nap too well or they seemed fussy, so you put them to bed early. This can sometimes mean that they have simply slept enough when

they wake or sleep pressure did not build enough before bed.

3. Learning a new skill. Developmental changes can mean that your baby starts practising these at night – rolling or crawling can be fun to practise in the cot. This is normally a short-lived phase. Try not to intervene if they are not upset.

4. They are ready for a nap transition. If your baby is ready to drop a nap but hasn't quite got there yet, it can sometimes cause a split night.

5. Unable to settle. As I have said above with early waking, if your little one doesn't get themselves to sleep, they are likely to find this even harder in the second half of the night. This is because there is less sleep pressure (see page 29). For example, if it is 3 or 4am, they might be tossing and turning for a long time until you step in. Then you might end up getting them up, playing and going to another room (all these things then stimulate baby), and so the cycle continues. They are then more tired the next day, and probably nap too long, and so we go on!

### To intervene or not?

If babies are happily playing, blowing raspberries, moaning or groaning, and seemingly calm, we need to leave them alone. We can rush to them when we think they are fully awake, when in fact they are just stirring between sleep cycles. If we do this, we can cause a long period of wakefulness in the night, while we continue the cycle of trying to get them back to sleep, when we really want them to be able to do it themselves. I've seen parents over the years who get their baby out of bed and watch TV and play downstairs (no judgement if you have done this), but it's perpetuating the cycle of periods of wakefulness at night. Try to keep things calm and quiet and stay in their room or your room if you can.

There is nothing wrong with attending to your baby at night, but sometimes we disturb them and stop them falling back to sleep.

## OVERTIREDNESS

It is understandable that we want to find a simple reason why our babies are not getting a settled night, and it's easy to use overtiredness as the scapegoat. It would be lovely to be able to tell you that, *yes*, it's because your baby is 'overtired'. Unfortunately, though, it's often just not the case. Sometimes we think the problem is that baby is overtired, but when we look at their overall sleep in 24 hours it is actually okay. Have a look at your baby and see if they are happy between naps, thriving and growing. If they are, then it's probably nothing to worry about. If they aren't, then look at the principles I cover in this book – routine, sleep environment and settling – to see if you can change something.

The fear of overtiredness can become a barrier to working on sleep. We get stuck on the never-ending merry-go-round of worrying about our baby's naps or sitting in a dark room trying to get them to nap.

We worry that by changing how we do things, baby could become even *more* overtired. The chances are you just need to follow their lead a bit more. Or you just need to mix it up a bit. Change the naps, change the bedtime . . . we need to change things to see the change.

Of course, we want age-appropriate naptimes and bedtimes, but each baby is an individual. Keeping them awake all day is a really bad idea, trust me, but also obsessing about forcing sleep is equally as bad. One person can only sleep so much in 24 hours. Often, I find that we feel exhausted ourselves and we assume that our babies are too.

I have honestly only ever seen a truly 'overtired' baby a handful of times in my practice, but they do exist. When a child is overtired, cortisol (the stress hormone) is released and it can make it hard to calm down – hence when you see little kids or babies who seem wired. If we have raised cortisol it can interfere with our sleep cycles and cause us to get less of the lovely restorative deep sleep stages (see page 28). This is sometimes why you'll see a fitful night or a very early morning after a long day out with fewer naps than usual.

If you are genuinely worried about this, take a step back. Maybe have a day out where you let all routine go out of the window. Let baby sleep when they need to – on you, in their buggy or in a sling. See what happens. Maybe they can tell you when they need to sleep? Maybe you will relax a bit and realise that it's not the end of the world if they appear tired. If they are taking a long time to get to sleep for naps and it's taking its toll, it's probably that they aren't ready yet. Pushing the time that they are comfortably awake, even by a little, can make a big difference. It is also always okay to give up on a nap, go and do a fun activity, feed or walk and return to the nap in a little while. If anything, I hope this book is going to give you the knowledge and confidence to do this and let go of the fear of overtiredness.

## NAP TRANSITIONS

It can feel hard to change things when you have settled into what feels like a good routine, but, as your little one grows and develops, they will need less sleep across the 24-hour period. A nap transition is when your baby drops one of their naps, perhaps going from three naps to two, or from two naps to one, and then eventually stops naps altogether. It can be difficult to navigate their changing sleep needs, but if you can keep on top of it then things should feel a bit smoother across the months and years.

Fewer, or no, naps means that although you have less time to yourself in theory, you do get more freedom to do fun things like baby groups and days out when your little one can stay awake and enjoy them.

There isn't an exact age or prescription for when they drop naps, and each baby will develop differently and have different sleep needs. It will also be influenced by what time they go to bed and their overall hours of night-time sleep. Therefore, it's often better to assess things across a 24-hour period.

Having said this, there are some common ages when babies often drop naps. I tend to say they drop to two naps between six and nine months, and down to one nap at around ten to fifteen months. If whatever you are doing is working and your little one is happy, you definitely don't need to change anything. However, if they are showing the following signs, it is worth looking at tweaking things before getting rid of a nap completely:

1. They won't settle for their nap anymore when they normally would. (This doesn't always mean they are ready to drop it, it might just mean you need to push it a little later or shorten it a little.)
2. They are waking up much earlier than usual from a nap, regularly (this can often happen for no apparent reason on occasion, so it is not always a sign!).
3. It could be that they nap fine but resist bedtime.
4. They might start waking up very early in the morning when they weren't previously.

Sometimes these things are just a sign that the nap needs to move a little or be cut a little shorter. You might also find that one day they seem to need the nap back, and then the next day they don't need it. Sleep needs to continue to fluctuate a little bit, especially across the course of a few weeks or even a month after they first show signs, before they are ready to drop a nap. It's always okay to add a nap back in if they seem to need it.

---

It's better to do things gradually if you can, rather than suddenly cutting out a nap altogether.

---

## MULTIPLES

Having twins or triplets doesn't mean that a settled night's sleep is out of the question. Of course, you have some added challenges, but logistically there is simply more planning involved!

Although your babies shared a womb, they are their own individual personalities – they don't always follow the same curve for many things, including sleep. This might mean that one twin (or multiple) sleeps better than the other(s). You can, however, get them on a similar routine in the day and hopefully get them sleeping well at night too, just as you would with a singleton.

There are a few ways to approach a sleep plan for multiple babies. If they share a room, you might find they sleep better in separate rooms (even if it is just a temporary measure), provided you have the space and they are over six months old. Having said this, I find most multiples sleep fine sharing a room, and you will be surprised how little their sibling wakes them.

It is often the case that one sibling is more sensitive than the other(s), so you can approach settling that baby first and then return to the other(s). White noise (see page 68) is a great solution as a tool to help your babies sleep well irrespective of whether their sibling is awake.

If you find it all too much of a juggle, you can try staggering their daytime routine by around 15 minutes or so. If you are caring for the babies on your own this might help you. As they grow and need fewer milk feeds during the day this should become much easier. Once they are on solids you will be doing mealtimes together anyway, which is so lovely.

It can feel lonely caring for any baby, but for parents of multiples in particular I highly recommend finding your local twins' group (see Useful Resources, page 283) for support and socialising. No one quite understands what it is to be a parent of multiples like other parents of multiples.

---

### *A triple plan*

*I once worked with a family who had triplets. Interestingly, one of the triplets was sleeping pretty well, but the other two were up every hour or two during the night. They were 11 months old when the parents got in touch with me. The triplets had had a very regular routine when they were five to six months old, but after they started solids and their sleep needs changed, things had gone a bit haywire. Mum and Dad were taking it in turns with the ever more constant wake-ups and giving them a formula feed almost each time. The wakeful triplets had very little appetite during the day. I discovered that they would have 200ml of milk at bedtime, and then 120–180ml at each night waking. We went through all of their history and, while they were born a little premature, they were hitting all the milestones of others their age, and size-wise they were all between the 40th and 50th centile (this is how a baby's size and weight is measured). Both Mum and Dad were tired (to say the least!) and really needed some help with more structure to their day and some more settled nights.*

*I reassured them that even though there were three babies to deal with, they had the same needs and we used all the same strategies that we would with a single baby. We looked at their bedroom first of all.*

*I recommended moving their cots a little further apart than they were – this was in the hope that they might not disturb each other as much as they had (although triplet 1, who slept a bit better than his siblings, was rarely woken by them). I soon discovered that he had dropped his morning nap and his siblings hadn't. Mum was worried this was too soon, but I explained that all babies have different sleep needs and some are ready to drop to one nap sooner than others. It was likely that his siblings still needed theirs as they were up so much at night (and he was generally up one to two times).*

*We decided to try a morning power nap on their way out to the baby group they went to (or the park or whatever activity they were doing that day). Mum had joined a fantastic group for other parents of multiple babies. They did a 15-minute nap in the car on the way, which meant they could get through to their next nap (after lunch) at home in their cots. Triplet 1 managed to get through without any morning nap at all. We worked on a great routine for the rest of the day (they didn't sleep again, having managed a long lunchtime nap) and started a new way of settling at bedtime. It turns out that usually Mum or Dad put down triplet 1 into his cot and he got himself to sleep, and they took another triplet each and fed them to sleep, or until they were sleepy, before putting them down. They were reliant on their bottles to get them to sleep, and to get them back to sleep during the night. They were going to turn one in three weeks' time, and I explained that very soon they wouldn't need formula or bottles anymore, and that solid food became a more important (and balanced) source of nutrition. In fact, triplet 2 had been suffering from constipation and their health visitor had suggested reducing her intake of formula.*

*We decided to go cold turkey on the night feeds. It felt like a big (and daunting!) change for them all, but the parents went for it. They put a chair in the triplets' room and took turns to comfort them. Triplets 2 and 3 did cry, but their parents supported them while they were in their cots. Triplet 2 was lifted out a few times for a cuddle, but they made it through to the morning. Lo and behold, the triplets ate a far better breakfast than usual. Within six days they were all sleeping through and taking one long nap at lunchtime, with an occasional power nap in the mornings. I explained that it was fine for this to vary day to day, according to their plans and how tired each triplet was.*

*Triplet 2's constipation got much better, and the triplets became much more adventurous with food. Just after 12 months they ditched their bottles entirely and had milk from a cup. The whole family was much more content, and the parents felt they could organise their days far better. Most important of all, they all got some well-needed rest at last!*

## TEETH CLEANING

This is an often-overlooked issue for many, and a puzzling question for others. I have been asked many times when we should start brushing baby's teeth and when to fit it into the bedtime routine. You should aim to start brushing your little one's teeth as soon as they come through. The timing of when their teeth will appear can really vary from baby to baby. When you're ready to begin, you can find age-appropriate toothbrushes and toothpastes in your local supermarket. You can also speak to your health visitor if unsure.

At first, it is all about getting them used to brushing and building it into your day somehow. Some babies will be reluctant to brush their teeth. It can help if you hold them or sit in front of a mirror so they can see what is happening. Also if you brush your teeth at the same time it can help encourage them to copy you. Eventually, we should be doing it twice a day – once sometime in the morning (ideally 20–30 minutes after breakfast) and once just before bed. You shouldn't rinse the toothpaste off, and it should ideally be the last thing that touches your baby's teeth at night.

Feeding from a bottle can cause cavities – whether it's breast milk, cow's milk or formula – because of the way milk pools in the mouth around the teeth. When breastfeeding, baby is actively sucking and swallowing when milk enters the mouth, so it's thought that milk directly from the breast doesn't pool like it does with a bottle. The possible exception to this is if baby has upper lip tie, which could potentially cause milk to pool around the teeth.

There is no proven link between breastfeeding and cavities, but breastfed babies can get cavities from other things, so it is still important to keep on top of teeth cleaning. If your little one does stay awake after their bedtime feed, it is worth adding teeth cleaning into your routine. Never give sugary drinks to your baby – they should only have water or their usual milk. Once your baby has teeth, you should start booking them regular trips to the dentist.

We should never leave our babies with their bottle in their cot for bedtime, as this means they are potentially sucking on their bottle teat very often, covering their teeth each time. Milk feeds should always be supervised by a parent, as otherwise there is also a risk of aspiration (choking on their milk). Not to mention you can cause your little one to reach for their bottle between every single sleep cycle potentially (as a method of settling themselves). This is a hard habit to break.

This can all feel difficult if your little one falls asleep on their bottle, but it can be a motivating factor for practising other ways of falling asleep. I advise keeping baby awake on their bottle where possible, and having a story, cuddle or lullaby before brushing their teeth 15–20 minutes later if you can. This might be hard on days when baby hasn't napped as long as normal or something else has disrupted your day. If there is a day when you aren't able to brush their teeth, don't beat yourself up but aim to try again the next day.

I really hope that the information on these topics is going to help you to future-proof your little one's sleep and to feel confident about these often puzzling topics. Remember, always listen to your gut and seek support if you need it. This support is likely to become even more necessary if you are returning to work, which I cover in the next chapter.

# 10

# GOING BACK TO WORK

The return to work after maternity or paternity leave can be daunting, even if you are in some ways looking forward to it. Your life as you've known it with your new baby is about to change and there is so much to consider.

You might be concerned about how you are going to go back to work on the little sleep you are getting if your baby isn't yet sleeping well through the night, or how you are going to manage a 6am start and caring for your baby, all before your 8am lengthy commute. You might have just got your baby sleeping well, or be in the process of doing so, and wonder how a new routine is going to affect that. It can be a difficult time for your baby too, forging new relationships with other caregivers and potentially spending periods of time outside of the home.

As with everything, you must do what works for you and benefits your family dynamic, so it is good to investigate all your options for childcare and, as part of that, how each setting might best meet your baby's sleep needs.

The tasks of getting ready for work, travelling to and from work and reconnecting with your baby after work can feel overwhelming. Taking things one step at a time and being really organised is key, as well as being confident in the childcare options you have selected so that you can go to work without the worry.

In this chapter I am going to cover the things to think about when choosing childcare, how to protect your little one's sleep and how to look after yourself when you return to work.

## YOUR FEELINGS

It is normal to feel totally torn and to experience guilt when you return to work. I find that, once you have a baby, there is always a push-pull between your duties as a parent and the rest of your life, whether that is a career, your social life or your other relationships. You are a parent now, and that is always going to be your priority. This means that you will always have thoughts of your baby in the back of your mind, even when you are in that board meeting, serving a customer, helping a patient or whatever it is that you do for work. You will always be wondering if they are napping okay without you or whether they are going to sleep well the night before a big meeting! But being a parent doesn't mean you can't continue to have a successful and enjoyable career. It can make it complicated at times, but with organisation and a good night's sleep, you can take on the world! You don't need to sacrifice every part of yourself to have a well-attached, happy child.

## THE TIMING OF SLEEP CHANGES

Going back to work is often a motivator for parents to take the step to work on sleep, but if you are thinking about making any big changes to how your little one sleeps, as detailed in Chapter 8, I would do this either in good time before your baby starts in their new childcare setting or after they are fully settled in. It is a big change in their lives to be away from you, so it's a lot to change everything at once. Having said that, there is nothing wrong with small, gentle changes at any time – like a regular bedtime routine for example . . . that is always going to be beneficial.

You might feel like you want to set your baby up to sleep independently in advance of them starting out somewhere new – maybe you want to improve night sleep so that the last months of your parental leave are well-slept. However, if, for example, you love your baby napping on you, don't feel that you need to change that in advance necessarily. Your baby will form new sleep associations with their new caregiver, and you might want to enjoy those last months of cuddling them on the sofa.

---

It can feel like an immense pressure to get sleep 'sorted' before your return, but don't stress out too much.

---

Give you and your baby lots of time to work on any changes to their sleep in advance of your return or surrender to it and know it will never be 'perfect', that you will still be able to function, even if it is on less sleep than you would like.

## CHOOSING CHILDCARE

This is the number one step, and arguably the most important. It can feel like a daunting task, but doing lots of research is key. You might choose childcare based on practicalities (such as location or opening hours), but it is important that you feel comfortable and safe with your choice. Depending on availability in your area and your personal preference (and let's not forget the huge financial implications), there are a few options to choose from. I am going to weigh up the pros and cons with your little one's sleep in mind.

First of all, when you choose a childcare provider, I urge you to ask lots of questions about their sleep policies.

Whoever is looking after your baby needs to know what you expect, and you need to know what they expect too.

### Nursery

At nursery your baby will be napping in a setting with other babies. It varies from nursery to nursery, but is often either a 'baby room' with cots or an area with mats – this could be part of the open room or it could be sectioned off. It is quite uncommon for these rooms or areas to be fully blacked out, but some will darken an area or corner of the space. When visiting prospective childcare settings, always ask to see the area where the babies will be napping. Some babies can become easily overstimulated with lots of noise and people around, so do bear this in mind. Think about how you feel in the settings that you are visiting – you might feel more relaxed in one than another which means your baby will probably feel the same.

Ask about their sleep policy:

- Do they have set naptimes for all the babies or will they follow your schedule?
- Will they wake babies if you ask them to cap a nap or do they have a no-wake policy?
- Will they allow comforters (see page 155)?
- Will they assist babies to sleep if they need it, for example, rocking, swaying, singing or walking to sleep in a pushchair?
- What would they do if your little one was resisting a nap?
- Do they insist on specific naptimes and, if so, what happens if your baby isn't tired at that time?

Remember, you are spending a lot of money and it is always okay to ask these questions.

Although your baby will be assigned a key worker, there may be times when that staff member is on a break, or off sick, or attending to another child. This means there is less continuity for your baby. In theory, their key worker is with them most of the time, so while it is not something to be too concerned about, it is worth considering if your baby is sensitive.

Most nurseries will have some outdoor spaces, so do check what they have available. Time outside during the day is important for your little one's body clock, their general well-being and for them to sleep well at night.

I have seen many babies over the years who happily nap in a light room at nursery, but need pitch black at home. Although I tend to recommend blackout for naps at home, it is not essential. Some babies nap perfectly fine with a bit of light. The same goes for noise – some will sleep soundly at a nursery with lots going on around them even if they need silence at home to stay sleeping. So, even if your baby is one who only sleeps at home in a quiet, dark room, they will likely surprise you with their adaptability.

### Mealtimes at nurseries

Nurseries tend to give 'tea' quite early – often at around 3.30pm. If this is the case, you'll need to make sure your baby or toddler has a snack when they get home, to prevent early waking due to hunger. Depending on what they have had at nursery, you might offer a sandwich, or some porridge or a banana and yoghurt when they get home, before their bedtime routine.

## Childminder

With a childminder, your baby might have their own space to nap or share it with one or two other babies or toddlers. There will likely be fewer other babies than at a nursery. Again, always ask to see the space where they will sleep and make sure you are clear about the ages and routines of the other children they are currently looking after.

A childminder setting tends to offer more of a 'home from home' environment. Childminders sometimes have more flexibility in terms of where your little one might sleep – for example, if they don't have other children to attend to, they might be able to take your baby for a walk to the local park or hold them to sleep. Do ask to see their garden or discuss how often they get outside.

A childminder will give you the continuity of the same person always looking after your baby. For some babies, this makes it an easier transition than nursery. As there are fewer babies around and a home-based environment, it also tends to be a quieter setting than a nursery.

The cons with choosing a childminder are that sometimes a childminder may be doing a school run for another child at a time when your baby is normally napping. They may also be juggling other babies or children (sometimes their own), so it's not always possible for them to be hands-on with settling. Again, it is important to ask them if they would be happy to wake your baby from a nap if you might want them to do this or what they would do if your little one resisted their nap. Most childminders will follow the routine you ask them to, but always check with them about this.

## Nanny

A nanny will care for your little one in your own home and replicate whatever it is that you do. The advantage of this is that your baby will sleep in their own bed and you don't have to worry about a drop off or the nanny splitting their attention with other babies (unless you are doing a nanny share of some sort). As the care is one-on-one, it can sometimes be easier for your baby to form an attachment and they don't have to share their carer with anyone else either. A nanny will do activities and take your little one out to playgroups, or whatever you ask them to do.

Always ask for references and the nanny's experience with sleep. Make sure your boundaries around sleep are clear, and let them know what you do and don't feel comfortable with them doing. Some nannies will also do overtime, which means that if you need to be back late from work or you work shifts they might do bedtime, or even babysit for you if you want to go out for the evening. It's nice to know that, if your little one was to wake while you are out, there's a friendly face to greet them.

The cons of employing a nanny are that they are generally more expensive than the other options and if you work from home and don't have a great deal of space, it can be tricky. However, if you have more than one child who needs care, it can work out to be cost-effective, especially if you have more than one at pre-school age.

### Family or friends

This is likely to be a much more affordable option (or even free in some cases with very willing family members or friends). Depending on your relationship with them and how well you communicate your wishes, they might follow your instructions and routine exactly or they might be fitting baby in around their own lives. In theory, you can have a bit more control over what happens with naps and routine, but I have also heard from many families over the years who have clashed with family members who won't follow their guidance and routine.

It can feel difficult and awkward to have conversations about your wishes if the childcare is free.

Communication and knowing where you all stand before embarking on the process is key here. Detailed instructions and a conversation with both you and your partner present can be helpful to put boundaries in place. Your family/friends might look after your little one in your own home or they might do it at their home. If they have baby at their home, you will need a spare cot or travel cot and highchair, for example. Make sure you are all okay with where baby will nap and your routine around this.

Bear in mind that there are some rules about registering as a childminder if your friend has your baby over a certain number of hours, so do check this. If you work nights or do shift work, you might need the flexibility of family and friends – some families do a mixture of more than one type of childcare. If this is you, make sure that your baby has a comforter/sleeping bag and, ideally, a similar routine is maintained. Writing down all of the information about your baby – such as routine and likes and dislikes – will come in useful here.

I explore more about handling relationships, especially with grandparents, in the next chapter.

---

Babies and children are very resilient, but when it comes to their sleep it is easier if the caregiver can follow your guidance. You are the parent; you know your little one best.

---

## FAMILIAR OBJECTS

A comforter (see page 155) is useful to help your baby settle when they are sleeping away from home. If they don't already have one, I would introduce it a few weeks in advance of starting childcare. This way it is a truly familiar and comforting item, rather than something 'new' that they just associate with their childcare setting.

If your baby doesn't have a comforter, consider a favourite toy that they play with in the daytime or anything that reminds them of home. You could even take an item of your clothing for them to hold and smell if they are unsettled and missing you. If you wear a particular perfume, you could spray some on a teddy!

Consider sending in their usual sleeping bag or one that has been slept in and smells of home. This is really reassuring for your baby when it comes to naptime. If you have a special or familiar book from home, you could send that with baby and ask their caregiver to read it to them before their nap.

## SETTLING-IN PERIOD

In most childcare settings you will be offered a 'settling-in' period. This means your little one spends short periods, or reduced hours, in their new childcare setting to get used to it. You should be offered sessions where you stay with them. This is a good way to get them used to their new environment. It is worth asking how many settling sessions they offer and what happens if your baby takes a bit longer to settle. Try not to worry if they don't nap as usual during this period.

It is really common for it to take some time for your baby to settle into their new surroundings enough to nap for as long as they usually do.

When you do leave after settling them in, it is important not to sneak off. Say an obvious goodbye, so that they know you are going. They will soon learn that you always come back at the end of the day. In preparation for this, and during your settling in period, I find games of peekaboo can help support the idea of separation from you.

## PROTECTING YOUR ROUTINE AND BOUNDARIES

You might have established a routine for your baby and feel concerned about protecting it and maintaining the settled nights that you currently have. It is important to communicate this to your baby's caregiver so that they understand your wishes. Ideally, they will be able to stick to what you do for naps, but if not then you might need to come to a happy medium. Be flexible, but also be forthcoming with your wishes and what is best for your baby.

It is quite common for little ones to struggle to nap for their usual length of time when they first start in a childcare setting. It is unfamiliar and it takes all of us time to build new habits. It is not uncommon for your baby to also take a shorter nap than normal. This can be down to the environment – the stimulation, the noise and being away from you and their usual routine – or it can also just be the fear of missing out on the fun!

If they have only had a short nap, you can adjust bedtime and try to put them to bed a little early, or perhaps they can have a short power nap on their way home. Try to avoid it being any longer than ten minutes or so if you can. If you are driving, opening a window, playing music and making sure your baby isn't overdressed can help to ensure they don't sleep for too long.

However, remember that it is okay to have a different routine to your usual routine at home on days where your baby is in childcare. Sometimes babies nap more on their days at home to catch up. You might also find that on the evenings that your baby has been away from you, they feed more if you are breastfeeding. This is for nutrition, but also connection. Don't rush your baby's bedtime routine. Take it slow, with lots of cuddles and eye contact.

If you are formula feeding, you may experience similar, especially if they have been less keen to have their normal milk with someone else. Whether they feed from the breast or bottle, our little ones connect with their primary caregiver. It can take time for them to accept milk from someone else, or any milk at all for some breastfed babies. You can try an open cup for milk if they won't take a bottle. If you usually feed to sleep, try not to worry – babies are very adept at creating new sleep associations for different people. They might feed to sleep for you, but be able to go down totally awake for someone else in a different location when they need to.

If they have a later or longer nap than at home, I really don't think it matters. It might feel alarming when you know that you stick to certain timings at home, but you can use this! Just adjust and give a later bedtime, giving you more time to reconnect with your baby once they are home.

It is okay to have a different routine to your usual routine at home on days where your baby is in childcare.

### Early riser

*I helped a mum once who was about to return to work. Her baby was nine months old and was waking two to three times per night (he would go back to sleep with some reassurance, but the wakings were quite regular). The problem was that, once she was awake, Mum struggled* to get back to sleep. She would be awake for hours potentially. She was really fearful about her return and wondering how on earth she was going to go back to work and concentrate. She was an anaesthetist and needed to really focus, for the sake of her patients, and her career.

I very quickly worked out what was going on. First of all, she was trying to put him to bed far too early. She had read (and been told) by various people that he would become 'overtired' if he wasn't asleep by 7pm at the latest. He was napping fairly regularly during the day (in fact he was still on three naps). There was no way he was ready for bed at 7pm, with the amount of daytime sleep he was having. We changed that straight off the bat and it immediately improved things. She liked to sit with him when he fell asleep and sing him a lullaby. I said that this was really lovely, and there was no reason that this couldn't continue. The real turning point was us realising that if he was going to sleep at 7pm, he needed to be awake from 2.30pm. In fact, some days he wasn't asleep until 7.15 or 7.30pm. With this longer wake window, he was much calmer and so was she, so this bred more calm!

She had found a lovely small nursery near their home, but was concerned about him napping there. He did have some hiccups for those first couple of weeks while he settled in, but before long she was astonished how well he slept there. He was a very active little baby, so was exhausted by naptime when he was there. The days when he hadn't napped as well, he did need an earlier bedtime, which I explained she shouldn't be afraid of. However, if he had napped well, then he needed to be awake for the afternoon in order to be ready for bed. In fact, the nursery had a 'no-wake' policy and a few days he slept for two-and-a-half hours at lunchtime. I advised that on these days she should put him to bed 10–15 minutes later than usual.

I explained to Mum that the return to work is a big shift, both physically and emotionally. We factored in time during her day when *she should sit quietly with a cup of tea or a book, or even have a bath and just be in silence. This helped her with her own sleep, and happiness too. Once they had both settled into their new routine, Mum was more relaxed and slept better herself (other than occasional night shifts at work, but that's another story!).*

**CHEAT SHEET**

Make sure that whoever is caring for your baby has a cheat sheet with lots of information on it. This could include:

- Notes on your baby's general routine.
- Food routine and likes and dislikes.
- Favourite activities and songs.
- Any emotional or behaviour cues, like sucking their thumb when tired, or any other obvious behaviours.

## ASSESSING YOUR BABY'S SLEEP

If you feel like your little one's sleep has really hit the skids since your return to work, it might be time to take a step back and reassess what is going on:

- Are they looking for more connection at bedtime because they are missing you?
- Are you rushing bedtime because you are tired?
- Have their sleep needs changed and their naps need tweaking?
- Have your bedtime boundaries moved? Are you doing something else you didn't do before?

If in doubt, start fresh with all the principles in this book: routine, sleep environment and settling. Don't rush bedtime, but also listen to your baby if they are tired. Working on all these things will help keep sleep in line, and make sure you are well-rested so you can function (see below).

## LOOKING AFTER YOUR OWN SLEEP

We spend all this time preparing our little ones for our return to work, that we sometimes neglect ourselves. My advice is to use their settling in period, and perhaps a few days of childcare, to prepare you for your return. Spend some time doing something nice (and don't feel guilty about it!), like getting a massage, going for a swim, buying new clothes or just doing something that you love. Have some time being you, in your own company. Get some early nights, and maybe even have some naps during the day. Maybe do some batch cooking so that you have some meals in the freezer for when you start work. Looking after yourself means that hopefully you will feel energised on your return to work.

Let's face it, once you are back at work there are going to be times when you are tired. It is sod's law that the day when you have a big meeting, are starting a new role or something else is going on, that is often when your baby will have a disturbed night. If you know you have something big or important on the next day, try not to get too anxious and fretful the night before. It is normal to toss and turn – I find taking time for myself to relax before bed helpful and, if your brain won't stop whirring at night, write it down. Sometimes journaling before bed can feel cathartic. It gives you some control and allows you to leave the to-do list for the morning, rather than having it flying around your brain when you are trying to get to sleep.

Try to get an early night when you can, but not too early (if we go to bed before we are tired it's a spell for getting frustrated and making it harder to sleep – we need that sleep pressure to build!). It can feel hard to commit time to unwinding after a long day at work and getting the baby to bed – you probably want to watch TV or scroll on your phone, but these things can sometimes stop us from going to bed when we would feel better the next day if we got an early night. Adding in some nice rituals that feel like a treat can help – reading a great new book, lighting a candle, wearing a silk eye mask or putting some new bedding on your bed . . . anything that will make bedtime a pleasurable draw for you. There are lots of apps on the market that can help with relaxation.

Don't put too much pressure on yourself to have everything 100 per cent perfect. No one can do everything, all the time. Parenting, working and looking after the home and ourselves can feel like spinning plates. If you drop one, don't feel bad – you are only human.

---

It can sometimes feel like a 'good' parent would be one who can do everything perfectly, but they simply don't exist. Good-enough is enough.

---

### Sharing the care

Let's also not forget your partner in this equation. Every family looks different and there may not be a co-parent, but for those who do have someone who shares parental duties, it is important to get them involved in the process too. If you can share drop-offs, pick-ups and bedtime routines, it feels a lot lighter. Often, I find that when the primary carer goes back to work, they end up maintaining all the primary care when they are at home, rather than sharing it with the other working parent. While for some families they have very clearly defined roles when it comes to domestic chores, it can feel like an easier transition back to work if you can explain to your partner that you don't have the time or capacity to do things as you did before. Hiring help where possible (even a cleaner once a month can take the edge off) or asking friends and family, and certainly communicating your needs to your partner, is key. It is always okay to let the people who love you know that you are struggling. I am going to talk lots more about this in the next chapter. It is always okay to reach out for professional help too.

### Getting through your work day

Returning to work is a big adjustment for you too and, even if your baby is sleeping well, you may not be getting the number of hours' sleep you had in your pre-baby days. You are also likely to be getting up earlier. Here are some practical tips for you to help you manage your work day:

1. Try to get out in the fresh air as often as possible. If you are in an office, try to sit by an open window.
2. Have regular movement breaks – even if this is a quick walk up and down some stairs, or some gentle stretching in the loo!
3. Eat regular, nutritious snacks for energy. Having some nuts, seeds and fruit on your desk is helpful – anything that is easy to grab.
4. Coffee can help in the short term, but don't overdo the caffeine and avoid having any after 2pm if you can, as it will negatively impact your sleep at night. You also don't want to get that horrible jittery feeling.
5. If you feel sleepy at work, try removing a layer of clothing. Being too warm is likely to make you want to nod off!
6. Hold off making any important decisions if you can. Save those for another day when you have had a bit more sleep.
7. Make sure you are drinking enough water. It sounds simple, but when we are dehydrated it can make us feel fatigued.

**8.** Once you get home, make sure you get an early night to catch up. Give that boxset a miss – as hard as it feels. I know you want some 'me' time, but you won't regret that early night tomorrow! If you aren't ready for bed and feel wired, try some gentle stretching, or read or listen to an audiobook or podcast. These things won't stimulate you like watching TV.

### Practicalities

When you have to get yourself to work (perhaps after little sleep), the mornings can be challenging. Giving yourself extra time to get ready is really helpful. Some parents find that if they get up before their baby, whether that's for a shower or a quick coffee, it can start the day off on a better foot. Or if you are making the most of every last wink of sleep, I'd advise organising everything the night before – lay out your clothes and your baby's clothes/bag. Practise your routine before you start back at work – work out what time everyone needs to be up, fed, dressed and out of the door for you to get to work on time. You might need to adjust your baby's routine to do this – perhaps a slightly earlier wake-up time might be necessary (as painful as that can feel!).

Try to be organised for when you get home with your little one. If you are picking them up from nursery or the childminder and it's going to be a rush through to bedtime, make sure you have a meal or snack available (if they haven't already eaten or need something extra) that is easy to prepare so that you can make the most of some nice connection time before bed. This can make bedtime far easier to navigate – they will want your undivided attention, even if it's just 10–15 minutes before you get into the bedtime routine. Obviously, if you finish work later than this it might not be possible (or if someone else is putting them to bed), but a bit of organisation here can give you a bit more flexibility so you can have an easier bedtime and more time overall with your baby.

Consider making a really easy breakfast the night before – I love overnight oats as the whole family can eat these. Setting the table for breakfast so that you have one less task to do in the morning can also be helpful.

Returning to work is a period of transition, like so much of parenting. I hope the advice in this chapter will help to make it easier for you.

In the next chapter we are going to look at another big change – your relationships with family and friends.

# 11

# SLEEP AND RELATIONSHIPS

When you have a baby everything changes. No matter how much you tell yourself that things will stay the same, your relationships with others will change and develop as you adjust to being a parent and embark on a brand-new relationship with your baby. In this chapter I am going to talk a little bit about some of the relationship issues that might occur, how sleep – or lack of it – could affect them and ways to support this seismic shift in your life, love and friendships.

## YOUR PARTNER

If you have a partner, I am assuming your relationship probably looks a little different to how it did before you had a baby. There is nothing that tests a relationship like the journey of parenthood, but your relationship doesn't have to suffer because of disturbed sleep. It's easy to forget one another and to focus purely on the baby, but your relationship is the foundation of your family. It deserves attention too. Relationships are like plants; we need to water them in order to grow.

### Sex

To point out the glaringly obvious, it's quite possible, and very common, for sex to be the very last thing on your mind when you have just had a baby. It made me laugh after the births of all my three children as almost the first thing that I was asked about by my midwife in the hospital was contraception. I was lying there sweating, with a baby hanging off my boob, so sex was the very last thing on my mind. (It is important to think about contraception when you are ready, though! Remember, while breastfeeding can affect when you ovulate, you can get pregnant while breastfeeding. This can happen before your period returns.)

You will be recovering physically and mentally from birth for some time and have hormones flying around your body, which can contribute to a low sex drive. And then there's the elephant – or, rather, your brand-new little baby – in the room. For some couples, it feels 'wrong' to be intimate while your baby is in the room. I can assure you that it will have no long-lasting effect on your blissfully unaware baby if they are in a safe sleep space and are loved and cared for. However, if you are bedsharing with your baby, this is when you need to get a bit creative with other rooms in the home.

Being ready for sex after having a baby is another thing and it should not be under duress or pressure from your partner. You might be tired if you are breastfeeding, or in fact whatever way you are feeding, and you might need some time without touching another person because you've had a baby attached to you all day. It's okay to not want to be intimate. But I do urge you to think about other ways of feeling loved and showing love in these times. Holding hands or hugging each other can go a long way during intense periods of sleep deprivation or adjustment to parenthood. Even sending a text to your partner when you are apart telling them you love them will help to keep a connection. To give and receive love doesn't have to be a physical act if you don't want it to be – 91 per cent of my followers on Instagram said they had less sex after having a baby when asked in a community poll. So, if you are feeling flat about your sex life, you are not alone.

We know from the latest research that the number of times we are woken in the night has a direct impact on our sex lives.[1] The more times you get up to settle your baby, the less satisfied you are with your sex life. This comes as no surprise, but it can be more complex than on first viewing. The wakings from your little one could be quite minor or they could be upsetting (depending on what is going on). We might just have less energy, we might feel underappreciated, but also there is a lot going on with our hormones after having a baby (if you are a birth parent) or if you are breastfeeding.

Some couples find that they get more sleep if they sleep separately. Some take it in turns with night feeds, while some have a set-up where one partner sleeps in a spare room to get some sleep. If you are not used to it, the physical distance from your partner can feel unnerving or you might feel like you get a better night's sleep and prefer it! Some parents have reported that they sleep better with just their baby in the room rather than their partner if they snore or move a lot in their sleep.

For some reason, it seems to be taboo, and awkward and embarrassing, for couples to sleep separately, even though many choose to do this. Even if you are sleeping separately right now, it doesn't mean it will always be this way. Intimacy will return, but it takes work. Laying the groundwork now with affection, and more importantly communication, is key.

For some couples, it works well to take the night shifts in turns. It's not always viable depending on who is doing the feeding (if your little one is exclusively breastfed it may feel impossible) and whether you have the space, but it's always worth trying to get your partner involved in winding, changing and settling baby even if they can't physically feed them.

For many parents, just feeling appreciated and cared for by their partner goes a long way. Sharing the load can also make it feel so much easier to cope with sleep deprivation.

## Communication

When we are tired, we are more likely to be short-tempered. We can also feel more emotional and underappreciated. This is where communication comes into its own. Learning to communicate your needs and feeling heard by your partner is key. Try sitting down in a quiet moment, perhaps while your little one is napping, and think about what it is you need from your partner. Making time for each other when your world has been turned upside down isn't easy, but trying to communicate in a calm manner when things are getting fraught is important. Remember that your partner is not a mind reader, and neither are you. Learning to communicate your needs out loud (which are just as valid as your baby's) is so important. We can get so caught up in making sure baby is napping, getting them to nap or managing their sleep and needs that we forget about our own.

## Teamwork

If you want to work on improving your baby's sleep, it is important to approach it as a team. Have clear boundaries and ideas on how you feel about sleep, and what steps you might take to improve it. What you do and don't feel comfortable with may look different, so try to find a middle ground. This is often the case with crying (please see Chapter 8). Discuss the methods in this book with your partner and between you think about which would best suit you as a family. Sometimes a discussion about your own childhoods and how sleep looked in your own families can be a useful exercise. Where do your beliefs about sleep come from?

Some things to think about (explore these ideas in a journal if you prefer) include:

- Where do your own beliefs around sleep come from?
- Did you sleep well as a child?
- What was your parents' attitude and approach to sleep?
- Did they ever tell you that you were a bad sleeper?
- Do your friends and family have babies who are 'bad sleepers'?
- What about your grandparents? Have they ever said anything about your parents' sleep?

Ideally, you and your partner should both do this exercise and then compare notes. How did considering the questions make you both feel? Did you discover anything new?

> These discussions are best held during daylight hours, rather than hushed arguments in the middle of the night while your baby is crying and stress levels are through the roof! A clear plan before you begin is better than a rushed decision and inconsistency at night-time.

Your sleep needs might be different to your partner's. If you need more sleep than your partner to function, practical solutions like them getting up with the baby in the morning while you catch up on sleep can make the world of difference.

It can be tricky if one parent is getting more sleep than the other. Perhaps you are breastfeeding and taking on all nights, or perhaps your partner works and you've decided between you that you will take the lion's share. Looking after your baby is also a job, a full-time job. You both need sleep to do your jobs, so coming to an agreement about the division of domestic chores, and sleep, can make things smoother. Having an honest but calm conversation – explaining that you are both doing a job, and that some support and recognition would make you feel valued and cared for – goes a long way.

There is, however, such a thing as competitive tiredness. So many couples argue about who got a worse night's sleep, whose turn it is to get up with the baby and who feels worse the next day. It is hard not to get drawn into a negative spiral here. Saying 'I am tired' does not mean that the other person is not tired. It's okay for you and your partner to say that you are tired.

---

It's okay to report to your partner how many times you were woken in the night, but it's better to use that energy to make a positive plan.

---

How could you approach things differently to support your family's sleep? Can you create a rota where you take it in turns to get up with baby? Even if your partner is working and you are at home, you still need to sleep. Perhaps you have decided that their sleep needs to be prioritised for them to work (which is entirely valid if that is how your family dynamic works), but even just knowing that on one or two mornings a week you get to catch up and have a lie-in can make the world of difference.

Perhaps you could treat it like a team at work – schedule in a 'team meeting' once a week, where both you and your partner talk about what is and isn't working for you, how you are feeling and any ideas about how you can reconnect if you are feeling that your connection is lost right now. Try to avoid criticising how they do things and use positive language when you talk about how you feel. If your partner isn't reading this book, perhaps show this chapter to them. Ask them to read it and then have a chat about how it made you both feel. Write down some notes and share them with one another.

You might find that you want to improve sleep, but your partner doesn't feel that there's value or doesn't agree with what you want to do. You both have a voice, regardless of who the main breadwinner or primary carer is. It's important that your needs are heard. If our car is broken, we take it to a mechanic, and sleep is no different. Using a sleep consultant or this book is not shameful. You have not failed and, if anything, it can improve your relationship and be beneficial for the entire family. Sometimes you need to be the person to stand up for yourself and explain – with love and respect – what you are doing.

Lack of sleep will test even the strongest of relationships. Don't ever make a rash decision when you are tired. When we are exhausted, we often don't pick up on subtle hints and behaviour changes in our partners, and vice versa. You might have the worst argument and then manage to have a nap and wake up feeling entirely different. Emotions can spiral out of control when we are tired and we might end up saying things that we don't really mean. It is worth acknowledging that and trying to resolve things when you are both a little less exhausted.

## SINGLE PARENTS

If you are a lone parent, I highly recommend getting a good friend or family member to stay with you in the early days and weeks after the birth, or you stay with them if you are living on your own. You will need time to rest, recover from the birth and adjust to being a parent. Don't be too shy to accept help whenever it is offered and ask for it when you need it. Instead of gifts of baby clothes and toys, consider asking for money towards expert help (see page 92). That room thermometer might be useful, but I know I'd have preferred a night off to something that isn't an essential item.

If you're dating you obviously need to have the time, the

finances and the energy to do that. Bad sleep can have a terrible impact on your feelings about dating or socialising in general.

If you have decided to work on improving your baby's sleep, enlist the help and moral support of friends or family. Speak to your ex-partner or co-parent about your plans, and make sure you are all on the same page. This is especially important if your baby sleeps at their home too. Trying to have an approach that is aligned with each other tends to be the most successful. If you don't have a good relationship or clash with them over the issue, you can continue to approach sleep in the way you like when your baby is with you. They soon understand the difference between different caregivers.

Some parents are very anxious that their ex-partner might do things differently, but as long as you are consistent with your baby when they are with you, it will be okay. This is where I highly recommend a comforter (see page 155) so that your little one has some consistency between homes – it smells familiar and can help them to relax when sleeping elsewhere. You can send a familiar story, toys and even a brand of baby wash for the bath for example.

We all value time to ourselves, but the single parent families I have helped over the years seem to feel this all the more. You need that time to yourself in the evening, as you are in charge and it's often harder for you to get a break. Those single parents who work for themselves need this time even more. Please don't feel guilty about prioritising yourself. It benefits the whole family for you to all be well-slept.

## FRIENDS

It is common to lose friends when you have a baby. Friendships you have had for years may drift apart and, if those friends don't have children of their own, it can be hard for them to understand what you are going through if you are sleep-deprived. It can be infuriating if your single friend without children tells you they are tired after you've had a long day, and an even longer night. Although everyone has the right to say they are tired, it can be jarring when you haven't had more than two hours' sleep in a row and haven't had a shower alone or a hot cup of tea in weeks.

You have less time than you had before, your finances might be stretched and you have a baby to care for. You also might find yourself choosing to sleep over socialising. This is very common! You are not alone if the thought of a night out fills you with dread. I think that redefining your friendships can be useful. Perhaps suggest a coffee date, a picnic or a lunch out where you can bring baby if you need to. Sharing with your friends is important – we need to know that they are going to support us when we need them, but we also need to work to maintain the friendships that we cherish. We might desperately want to go out and do the things we used to do, but, in the early days especially, it can feel difficult to even think about. There will come a time, I promise, when you are all sleeping better and you will be ready to go out and see your friends. If you are honest and tell your friends you are struggling, then the good ones will understand.

Friendships change and evolve and that's okay. Sleep can play a part in how we interact with our friends, how we socialise with them and where we forge our new friendships. A good friend will hopefully pick up the phone when you call them for a chat and take the time to understand what you are going through.

It's okay to prioritise your sleep, and health, at the expense of a friend who doesn't quite get it.

### Avoiding comparisons

You may have friends who are parents who do things differently to you or who approach their little one's sleep differently. This can feel quite jarring, especially if they give you advice that you didn't ask for or that feels at odds with how you approach things. It is important to remember the other things that you like about your friend and try to avoid conversations about how well your baby is sleeping if their baby isn't sleeping well, and vice versa. It's hard not to compare babies, especially if they are of a similar age. It's okay to do things differently to how your friends do things – it doesn't mean that you don't have anything else in common. It can be hard not to compare to those parents we see on social media too – remember they are showing us a highlight reel.

### New friendships

Hopefully you might find new friends too – whether that's from an antenatal group, or a baby class, or someone you meet at a local cafe. The early days with a new baby are certainly not easy, and it can feel very lonely, especially if you are tired. Having a regular routine with your baby as they grow will put you in good stead for going to these classes and socialising. It means you can predict roughly when they will be tired or hungry, and plan around this. No one wants to go to a baby class with a cranky baby (although you certainly won't be alone if you do).

## RELATIONSHIP WITH YOUR BABY

The most unique, earth-shattering, exciting and tiring relationship you will ever have is with your baby. Not everyone feels that rush of love immediately, and that's okay. Like any relationship, it can feel strained if you are not sleeping well. As much as you love your baby, it is okay to say you are struggling – it doesn't mean you love them any less. You wouldn't be expected to do any other job where you were woken multiple times in the night and had no breaks and no holiday. It's not easy. It can be joyous, but it's not easy.

Bonding with your baby and getting to know them takes time – just like any other relationship. And let's remember, if you're the birth parent, you are undergoing a huge physical change – recovering from birth, whatever that looked like. You might have been awake every hour since your baby was born – let's face it, it's not the most ideal situation for a brand-new relationship, but we move with it. This is why support is so important. Your partner, friends or family being there so that you can take a nap, however short, to give you some space to rest and be in a good place to enjoy your baby is invaluable.

As your baby grows and you start to work on sleep, you might find yourself getting frustrated with your baby. This is also normal and shouldn't be a taboo. Just because you feel annoyed in the moment, it doesn't mean you don't love your baby.

---

It is okay to not love being woken through the night.
It is okay to find it hard and, for some, the hardest
thing they have ever done.

---

Remember in those moments to take a deep breath – if you need to, step out of the room. It's better to take a moment to collect yourself than express any anger or frustration towards your baby. Make sure they are safe and give yourself a moment.

Like any relationship, your relationship with your baby grows, fluctuates and changes over time. We have blissful times, and hard times, and dark times. If you can get a little more sleep then I hope that things will seem brighter, easier and more joyful. The beautiful little person who might feel like a stranger at first will become your best friend later.

## *No comparison*

*I met a mum, Sarah, who had a baby just two weeks after her best friend, Rebecca. They were both first-time mums. Rebecca's baby had seemingly 'slept through' the night from the very early weeks, whereas Sarah's baby had been very wakeful. Sarah had introduced a dummy (even though she wasn't keen on the idea), just to help comfort her baby a little. He'd had 'colic', which in fact turned out to be a cow's milk allergy, and had had some really tough early weeks and months. Sarah had really struggled as, although Rebecca was sympathetic, she just couldn't understand what Sarah had been going through.*

*Rebecca had taken to breastfeeding like a duck to water, and Sarah had really struggled and switched to formula in the first week. They had confided in one another, but it seemed that the comparisons started drawing in — from friends and family, and each other. Rebecca had tried to give Sarah advice, which just didn't suit her baby. She needed to be hands-on with him, as he had had such a tricky start. He wasn't calm if she 'just laid him down'.*

*We worked on a super gradual plan together when he turned six months. He needed her support at every sleep time, and she was okay with that. The breakthrough for Sarah was when he slept for a few hours in the evening for the very first time, without being held. For her, this was a triumph. She ate a meal in peace with her partner. We kept his dummy as it wasn't causing any extra issues for him. Sarah would replace it each time she comforted him during the night. We reduced his night wakings from six to seven times to only one to three. On many nights it was just one. This might not have been the same as Rebecca's baby, who slept from 7pm until 7am, but I explained how babies are all different and, while it wasn't 'perfect', her baby had come on leaps and bounds from where he was. Comparison really is the thief of joy. It turns out that Rebecca had been really struggling with postnatal anxiety, and in fact hadn't been coping as well as she had appeared to be. Thankfully, the friendship lasted, and they found other things to talk about, not just sleep!*

## INTRUSIVE THOUGHTS

When you are sleep-deprived, you might have some dark thoughts. It's pretty taboo to talk about, but 'intrusive thoughts' are common. This is when something awful pops into your mind – an image or a thought about harm to your baby, for example. Talking about these thoughts and understanding that you aren't going to act on them, and that they are not real or harmful, can be helpful. Remember – a thought is just a thought. I want you to know that other people experience these too. We don't really know why, but looking after this small person who is entirely dependent on you means you are in a high state of alert. We are designed to worry about their safety. Any kind of anxiety is worsened by sleep deprivation, so do be mindful of prioritising your rest, and getting help wherever possible.

If you are struggling with this, please seek professional support from your GP, or a referral to a psychology service if you need it. If you feel like you might actually harm your baby, please call 999 (in the UK), visit the accident and emergency department or call the Samaritans on 116 123.

## GRANDPARENTS AND OTHER 'ADVICE-GIVERS'

Countless families have mentioned conflict to me with their family over the years, most often with grandparents – differences of opinion, unsolicited advice and generally clashing on conversations and approaches to sleep. First, I am not bashing grandparents. They can be the most loving, caring and nurturing influences if you are lucky enough to have them in your baby's life. They can also be a vital lifeline.

Maybe you have your own parent or your partner's parent who is an amazing support, but it is not always easy to navigate the changes in your relationship when a baby arrives and you need to communicate your own beliefs and needs. The whole dynamic of your family shifts when there is a new person to factor in. Your parents or your partner's parents might have their own preconceived views about how baby should sleep, whether they should be breast- or bottle-fed, whether you should return to work and so on and so forth. It is worth noting that what they did with their babies was some years ago. Not only has advice and research moved on since then, but it is okay for you to want to do things differently. Equally, what they say might be really reassuring and helpful – we can't assume all advice is outdated. Remember that, no matter how strained things are, they have your best interests at heart.

---

It is okay to establish boundaries and to stick to them. The tricky (and important) part is how you communicate them.

---

Communicating your wishes and boundaries is sensitive sometimes. When it comes to in-laws in particular, I advise having a conversation with both you and your partner present. Sometimes it is easier if your partner explains what you are doing, or what you would like them to do (if they are helping with baby), or the expectations if you have a family occasion, for example. See page 44 for advice on how to approach any aspect of baby care with grandparents.

I can give some extreme examples of things that I have heard over the years – parents having to explain why we don't give rusks in bottles anymore or how babies should be laid down to sleep on their backs. We have evidence, and we know better now, so we do better. Some older relatives might say things like, 'It didn't do you any harm', but just because you turned out okay, it doesn't mean that the practices were the best thing for you. When my older brother and sister were little, we had no law in the UK that we had to wear a seatbelt (in fact, it came in when I was about six months old). Just because we survived, that doesn't mean that no seatbelt was a great idea. Your grandma might have dipped your mum's dummy in whisky, but we know now that's a bad idea!

You may have the same experiences with other family members – aunties, uncles, siblings, cousins . . . and even random strangers in the supermarket! The list goes on. It can feel hard to stick to your guns if you have been used to 'people-pleasing' and not wanting to rock the boat. Parenthood really can be a shift in mindset, and your needs are so important. Don't forget that.

We know that all babies are different, but some families face challenges that they might not have been expecting, or babies who need a little more care. So next up I have included some advice for those who need it.

# 12

# SPECIAL CONSIDERATIONS

In this chapter I cover some special circumstances that require sleep support to be tweaked and tailored. It is by no means comprehensive, but I have chosen some of the conditions I have worked with personally and am qualified to advise on. Please remember this is not a substitute for professional medical advice, diagnosis or treatment. If you are ever worried or concerned about your baby, always speak to a medical professional.

## PREMATURE BABIES

All the sleep advice I have given in this book applies to premature babies too, but it may take them a little longer than a full-term baby to 'sleep through'. Having said this, you will find that your newborn will likely spend a lot of time sleeping over a 24-hour period but wake regularly for night feeds. Overall, they spend less time in a deep sleep compared to full-term babies, and it might seem like they never 'fully' wake up. This will change over time as they grow and catch up with their contemporaries.

Many parents of premature babies ask me if they should go by their baby's actual or corrected age (see box below) when considering sleep training. It is very individual to your baby and their development, but I tend to go on corrected age to be cautious. As I always say, though, you can absolutely try working on routine, sleep environment and settling (the gentle end of the scale) at any time.

## HOW TO WORK OUT CORRECTED AGE

Start with your baby's age in weeks or months since they were born. Subtract the number of weeks premature they were born. So, if your baby was born 4 weeks early and is now 24 weeks old, their corrected age would be 20 weeks (5 months old) and it could be that they aren't ready for sleep training until they are 7 months old. Similarly, if they were born 8 weeks early, they might not be ready until they are 8 months old.

### Sleep safety

Premature babies are more vulnerable to SIDS (see page 50). In a neonatal unit, they may have slept on their front or with rolled-up towels to keep them in position. Once they are home, you need to follow safe sleep guidelines (see page 51) and place them on their back to sleep.

Be mindful that a sleeping bag may not be appropriate for a premature baby if they don't come in a small enough size (always check the weight guidance), so a well-tucked-in blanket with your baby's feet at the foot of the cot (make sure the blanket only reaches your baby's shoulders and can't cover their head) or a swaddle (see page 56) is fine. You might find that it's a big period of adjustment to sleep at home, after having been in the hospital.

Your baby might have worn a hat in the hospital, but at home they don't need one anymore. It is important that babies don't overheat as it is a SIDS risk. It's also not recommended to co-sleep with a premature baby. Premature babies are more vulnerable to infection so try to keep visitors and pets away from their sleep space and keep it clean.

## PARTIALLY HEARING AND DEAF BABIES

I have helped several partially hearing and deaf babies to sleep well over the years. The basics are the same, but there are some adjustments and things to consider.

A partially hearing or deaf baby will only be soothed vocally if they are lying on you, so that they can feel the vibrations of your voice from your chest as you talk to them or sing a lullaby. Or if you hold them cheek to cheek as you talk, they can feel the rhythm of your voice. All of these activities can form a lovely part of a bedtime routine.

If one of our senses is not as strong as the other, the other senses can be heightened. This means that for deaf or partially hearing babies, loving touch can have an even more powerful impact. I recommend baby massage (see page 115) as it is relaxing and signals the approach of bedtime. This physical touch can be incredibly calming and creates oxytocin, the love hormone that promotes sleep. Cortisol, the stress hormone, is also reduced, which is really useful to help a baby to relax in the lead up to bedtime.

When you blackout the bedroom for a partially hearing or deaf baby, you remove one of the senses they rely on – sight – and this can leave them feeling a little disorientated. For this reason, I recommend a night light, from babyhood. I would introduce one with an orange, amber, red or pink colour as these are sleep-friendly colours. The alternative would be leaving a light on outside their room, and not closing their bedroom door. You can also try glow-in-the-dark stickers on the ceiling – this can become a familiar reassurance. Of course, some babies will be fine in a dark room, but I have observed in my practice this can make a big difference in supporting sleep.

A comforter is fantastic for deaf babies, as they use their sense of smell and touch (as all babies do), but for some these senses can be heightened, especially at bedtime when they are trying to calm down and relax for sleep. Make sure you are following safe sleep guidelines around comforters (see page 155).

### Settling methods adaptations

If you are comforting your partially hearing or deaf baby in their cot as part of one of the sleep methods (see Chapter 8), you can try placing your hand on them, stroking their head or face, or patting their bottom (if they are sleeping on their front and are old enough to roll both ways). You can also try tapping the mattress close to them so that they feel the vibrations. It is important to use some touch or vibration. I have even known parents to hum on their baby's stomach.

If you have a small baby, swaddling or tucking them in well if you use blankets (which is part of safe sleep guidance anyway) can be really helpful.

> For parents who are partially hearing or deaf, there are flashing and vibrating monitors that alert you when your baby is crying.

## PARTIALLY SIGHTED AND BLIND BABIES

Babies who are partially sighted or blind can encounter some challenges with sleep due to their perception of light and dark. It is tricky for them to control their internal body clock (circadian rhythm) with limited light. This also affects the production of melatonin, which lets your body know that it is night-time and signals it to relax and fall asleep.

Focusing on a very regular routine is key with blindness to

ensure your baby isn't sleeping too much during the day. If they are at the age when they are eating solids, having regular meal-times will help to establish a daytime routine.

Making the bedtime routine as relaxing and sensory as pos-sible is helpful. Use strong verbal and physical cues as you do things. Even for smaller babies, start telling them, 'It is night-time now' or 'It is bedtime now.' If your baby doesn't see, they will still know that night-time is coming with your verbal cues and the familiar sounds and smells of their routine.

You can add in physical activities such as baby massage or per-haps brushing their hair or kissing their neck. Using scented bath wash or soap can make bedtime a fun experience, and scent can be a powerful cue for all babies. You could use toys in the bath that make interesting noises too. Touching their favourite soft toy or teddy while you read a familiar story is good to include in your baby's bedtime routine too.

Those who are visually impaired but have some sight can still be disturbed by light coming into their room or the glare from screens or polished surfaces. Always cover these if possible. You can try having contrasting colours in their room – furniture, bean-bags and toys. This can help make their sleep space recognisable and familiar.

When working on a sleep plan, be sure to choose a verbal cue – such as 'night night'. When you are reassuring your baby, try to use the same cue each time. Placing your hands on them, sshing, pat-ting or holding can be effective.

Everyday speech and language is good for all babies and their development, but is even more important for a visu-ally impaired child to help them start to distinguish when they have changed location or are going to change loca-tion. Don't feel silly about explaining things to your baby – you are teaching them about their home and the world around them. Start addressing your baby by their name quite early on – this means that, as they grow, they will recognise it, and therefore not miss things that are directed at them.

## HIP DYSPLASIA

Hip dysplasia or DDH (developmental dysplasia of the hip) is a condition in which the joint of the hip doesn't properly form. It can affect one or both hips and is more common in girls.

A baby's hips should be checked within 72 hours of them being born. Your baby would be referred for an ultrasound at between four and six weeks old if there are any concerns about the hips, if there is a history of childhood hip problems in the family or if your baby was breech at or after 36 weeks' gestation.

If a baby is diagnosed with DDH, they are usually treated with a Pavlik harness. This works by keeping both hips in a stable position so that they can develop normally. This harness tends to be worn across several weeks and will be fitted and removed by a health professional. They will give you information on how to change baby without taking it off and how to position baby when they are sleeping.

It can feel hard and alarming to have your baby in a harness, but they will get used to it. All the usual sleep guidance applies, but it is normal for a baby with hip dysplasia to need much more support from you when they are falling asleep while they are getting used to their harness (the first two to three nights tend to be the trickiest). It might be that you need to rock them or sit with them or cuddle them to get them to go off to sleep. Regardless, you can absolutely benefit from a routine. You want that lovely sleep pressure to build before you try to settle them to sleep, otherwise your baby is likely to get more upset. This won't be forever, and you can work towards independent sleep later if you like. Most babies adapt very quickly and sleep well with their harness.

Practical tips for settling babies with DDH:

- Always place your baby on their back while they sleep.
- The harness might irritate their skin – you can wrap some soft material around the bands if this is the case. Some families find that longer toddler socks can provide some extra protection. You can ask your clinician for advice on removing the harness for short periods if possible.
- You can try a designed-for-purpose sleeping bag or swaddle – some high-street brands now have a range with a wider fit at the bottom to allow for a harness or brace. You can also find clothing made to fit around a harness.
- Always keep an eye on your baby's temperature – for a true gauge, feel their chest or the back of their neck. If they are wearing a harness and the weather is very hot, it's okay for them to just sleep in a nappy.
- Some families will roll up a towel or blanket and place it under their baby's knees. This should only be done under the advice of your clinician, so do ask them if you are unsure.
- Sometimes, due to the lack of movement in the hip, there can be some tension in the pelvis that leads to colicky symptoms. If your little one suddenly starts to show these signs and struggles with their digestion, then try to include some gentle baby massage on the tummy in your daily routine. Always rub gently in a clockwise direction, taking care not to put pressure on the bladder. Sometimes due to the lack of movement in the hip there can be some tension in the pelvis. This can be helped by baby massage yourself, or seeing a paediatric chiropractor or osteopath could be helpful.

There is also a cast called a hip spica that is used if your little one has had surgery on their hips. You should always place your baby on their back to sleep and follow the advice I have given above. If you are ever unsure, always consult your clinician. I have also added some Facebook pages to the Useful Resources section on page 283 about hip spica, which can be a great support to parents.

## TALIPES (CLUB FOOT)

This is when the foot points down and the sole of the foot faces backwards. Treatment involves manipulation of the feet, a plaster cast to correct it over time and eventually boots and a bar. The boots and bar keep the feet in position, which stops the muscles and ligaments from returning to their old patterns.

Practical tips for settling babies with talipes:

- Footless sleepsuits are essential. A sleeping bag is helpful so that your baby doesn't get tangled up in blankets.
- Your baby may end up in some funny sleeping positions, but try not to worry. If they are uncomfortable, they will let you know. Be mindful of their temperature as always and adjust their clothing appropriately.
- If your baby wears boots and a bar and suddenly starts waking very often, it is worth checking the distance between the boots is still shoulder-width apart. As your little one grows, the bar will need to be widened. Also check for any blisters or rubbing – this can obviously cause discomfort, especially at night-time. (Do speak to your physiotherapy team about both of these things.)
- Casts and boots are unlikely to cause your baby pain, but they do often cause frustration. This is normal, and it can take time for them to get used to the feeling.

- Your baby can sleep in their own sleep space or you can follow safe co-sleeping guidance if that works better for your family – make sure there is no loose bedding or pillows near them and refer to the general safe sleeping guidelines too (see page 51).

## REFLUX

If your baby has reflux and it is unresolved and untreated, I wouldn't embark on sleep training. You can, however, still benefit from working on a good rhythm to your day, and sleep environment. It generally works better to wait until you are confident your little one is comfortable before working on changing how they fall asleep.

It is always good to be curious about reflux (see page 88) and see if you can get to the bottom of what is causing it. Always get a feeding assessment and skilled feeding support where possible and think about the following things:

1. Is my baby tongue-tied? If so, it can cause excess air when baby can't get a deep latch on breast or bottle. You can ask a feeding specialist to check this for you.
2. Check your baby's latch – are they getting a good mouthful of breast? If bottle-feeding, are they able to form a seal around their bottle?
3. It can be worth experimenting with different bottles – there's no need to buy every brand, but sometimes a different shaped teat can help.
4. Are you formula feeding and shaking the bottle to mix it up? It is better to swill it gently and stir with a sterilised spoon if the formula has not dissolved properly. The excess air created from shaking will cause your baby to reflux.
5. Speak to your health visitor or doctor about a potential course of action. It is important to get support.

6. If you think your baby might benefit, you can try seeing a paediatric chiropractor or osteopath to check whether there is any tension in their body that is causing problems when feeding.

7. Try feeding your baby in a more upright position.

8. If you are formula feeding, be careful not to overfeed. You might find that smaller, more regular feeds are helpful. Some of my clients with reflux babies find it useful to do a split feed at bedtime – half the feed before the bath and the other half afterwards.

9. Make sure you wind your baby after feeding. Wind can sometimes get stuck at the top of the stomach. Holding them and tilting them slightly to their left-hand side can be very effective – this works with the direction of their stomach as the opening is slightly over on the right-hand side.

10. Hold your baby upright for 20–30 minutes post feed. You can try walking around and singing a lullaby or saying goodnight to toys and teddies.

11. Wear your baby in a sling during the day – if your reflux baby won't settle for naps in their cot, it is not a problem. It is better that they get some rest and you have your hands free, than you spending long periods of time trying to get them down when they are in pain.

## ECZEMA

Eczema is uncomfortable and can cause sleep disruption. If your baby is itchy, it can wake them up or make it hard for them to feel comfortable to sleep. Speak to your doctor for a course of action to get the eczema under control. This might include keeping a diary of potential triggers. You might be referred to a dermatologist.

Some practitioners will advise daily bathing, while others suggest every few days – it really depends on your baby. If you want to have a consistent bedtime routine without bathing every day, I suggest taking your baby to the bathroom regardless and washing their hands and face, and changing their nappy and sleepsuit. This way they still have the physical change of room, and it can help them prepare for bedtime as they learn the order of what happens at the end of their day.

It is always important to be mindful of your little one's temperature, but becoming overheated can really aggravate eczema. Dressing your baby in soft cotton is a good idea as it is breathable and kind on the skin. Any rough or synthetic materials can exacerbate things. You can also use mittens on your baby's hands to stop them scratching.

Make sure your little one's eczema is under control before considering any controlled crying, but you could absolutely try some of the slow, gentle methods outlined in this book.

## ALLERGIES

### Cow's milk allergy

This can cause pain, bloating and diarrhoea, which can, in turn, quite understandably, have a big impact on sleep. Once the allergy is confirmed, your doctor might prescribe you a formula, or if you are breastfeeding you will be advised to remove dairy from your diet. Once the allergen has been removed, your baby should start sleeping more soundly within a few weeks or so. You should only do this under medical advice. It is a big thing to change if you aren't sure that your little one has a cow's milk allergy. Who wants to give up chocolate and cheese if they don't have to?! This is why it is always worth having a proper assessment and diagnosis with your doctor or a paediatric dietician first.

### Other food allergies

Of course, there are other foods that your little one can be allergic to and, before you become aware of this, it could affect their sleep and potentially become an emergency situation. For this reason, I recommend introducing common allergens earlier in the day when you are introducing new solid foods. This means you will be able to observe your baby carefully, rather than any reaction happening in the middle of the night. If you have a family history of allergies, it is worth being particularly careful.

Common foods that can trigger an allergic reaction include:

- cow's milk
- eggs
- foods containing gluten (wheat, barley and rye)
- nuts and peanuts (we should only serve these to babies crushed, ground or as nut butters)
- seeds (also crushed or ground)
- soya
- shellfish (only serve cooked)
- fish

These foods can all be introduced at around six months old when you are weaning your baby.

### Dust mites

Some babies, children and adults can be allergic to dust mites. These are tiny, invisible creatures that live in everyone's home, in spite of regular cleaning. They are often found in bedding, mattresses and soft toys. Common symptoms of an allergy could be sneezing, coughing, watery eyes and a runny nose, or they can be a trigger for eczema or asthma attacks. These symptoms would be worse at night.

Things you can do to help your baby:

- Wash bedding frequently, at a high temperature.
- Vacuum regularly (for severe allergies a wooden floor or vinyl can be better than carpet).

- Choose curtains that can be washed or blinds that can be wiped.
- We don't want to stop your baby from having a favourite soft toy or comforter, but try to keep them to a minimum (one or two favourites, for example). You should aim to wash or freeze them at least once a month. The process of freezing them kills the dust mites.
- 'Damp dusting' can help too.

## ANY OTHER CONCERNS

If your baby is diagnosed with any condition or has any other physical challenge in their life, it is possible that it can affect their sleep. Given that sleep is linked to every system in the body, this is no surprise. Ask your healthcare practitioner for advice on sleep when you are gathering information about your child's condition or when you are discharged from their care. They may well have a fountain of knowledge on how you can adjust sleeping conditions or some handy tips or tricks you can use. It is always okay to ask.

Everyone deserves a good night's sleep, but it can be a bit more challenging for some than others. Don't give up and seek support, whether that's professional or whether you enlist friends and family to support you, while you support your child.

# CONCLUSION

Well, that was a ride, and I hope you have enjoyed it as much as I enjoyed writing it for you. Refer back to page 17 where I asked you to think about your attitude to sleep to see how far you have come, and also to work out if your thoughts and feelings around sleep have shifted. Perhaps you have tried things and they have worked, perhaps your goalposts have moved. Make notes again if it's helpful – you could even write a letter to yourself to read when you are struggling. We can be our biggest critics, but if we tune into our innate wisdom, we often give ourselves the best advice.

We have covered every possible twist and turn of your little one's sleep journey. From the early days to the blips in sleep, the 'regressions', your relationships and going back to work. This is real life that you are living beyond the pages of this book – it is never going to be perfect, no matter how closely you follow my advice. But you are a good parent. You are a parent who cares enough to have taken the time to read this book and to make it all the way to the end (thanks for sticking with me). No matter how hard we strive for it, perfection doesn't exist – whether that's in our actions, parenting in general or sleep. There is no perfect baby, but there is *your* baby, who you know best, who loves you best and who you are made for.

I want to thank you for trusting in me to be the one to educate you on the topic of sleep. There are so many voices out there, so thank you for choosing me. I want to set your baby up with great foundations for sleep, for the rest of their life (and your life!). We can only do the best with what we have, and now you have a book full of knowledge around sleep. I truly owe thanks to all the families who I have helped over the years – each baby and each family taught me something new. I am honoured to be passing this knowledge on to you and to others to help shape the sleep of future generations.

The world keeps turning and things keep changing, and I feel like there is real progress on the horizon. I hope that in the coming years it becomes normalised to seek sleep support, without shame and guilt, and commonplace to talk about the ups and downs with our peers. I really hope that you can have it all – a baby who sleeps, a career, a good relationship and your health. There will be challenges ahead, but hopefully you will be well-slept enough to face them head-on.

## You deserve the best.

I really hope that this book has armed you with the practical tools to be your own expert. While the world can feel narrower when we become a parent, I want to give you options and choices to widen your horizon. You know, there really is no secret sauce, but there are a whole lot of things you can try, if you want to. It's not easy and can take hard work, consistency and a lot of soul-searching, but we can find the path that feels right for us, and for our babies. We all have entirely unique priorities, experiences and family dynamics to consider. What is right for one person is wrong for another. We just need to have options and be confident that whichever path we choose is the right one for our families.

Good sleep shouldn't be reserved just for those who are 'lucky' to have a baby who is laid back, nor should it be for those rich enough to have a nanny to do the hard work for them. Regular, normal people should have access to good-quality sleep support. I hope that this book makes waves; that it lights a fire inside you to prioritise your basic needs and to live your life to the fullest.

The topic of baby sleep can be so divisive and so many people tell us what we should and shouldn't be doing with our babies. We all have our own important needs and unique style of parenting. You can always find your own style or pick bits from what you see and what you like. You know your baby best, but please don't ever be afraid to ask for help or tell someone you are struggling. Parenting is not an easy job, and it's even harder on little sleep. You are normal if you don't enjoy every second, so please don't feel guilty. You are not weak, you are brave! Make peace with the choices you make. You make them for a good reason – don't doubt your intuition.

---

Every day we learn and grow as parents, just as our babies learn and grow.

---

We go through phases in our lives, just as our babies go through phases in theirs. Some of them will be more challenging and some will feel easy to navigate. Don't be afraid of failure – you are your baby's safe foundation who they can always return to. Your loving boundaries and your care, time and commitment will pay dividends in the long run. Even if it doesn't feel like it at times, there is always hope just around the corner. Enjoy their babyhood, for what it is. It's beautifully imperfect, it's messy, it's chaotic, but you blink and you'll miss it.

This truly is the book that I wish I had had when I had my first baby, and I hope that it is just the companion that you need. I hope it becomes weathered and dog-eared, underlined and scribbled in. Much like a well-loved recipe book, the recipe to a good night's sleep is hard to find. You now have the tools to change your life, rewrite your story and find your way out of the darkest corners of sleep deprivation. It can be so dark on those long, lonely nights, but you are not alone. Across the world there are other parents doing the very same thing, in the very same moment as you. I hope that, if nothing else, this book can bring you light, make you feel less alone, give you hope and peace, and ultimately the good night's sleep that you deserve.

# PROBLEM-SOLVING QUESTIONS AND ANSWERS

This section includes real-life questions and answers from some of the parents I have helped. I hope it will give you some ideas of tweaks you can make, and answers to questions you may have.

### Q: When will my baby sleep through the night?

**A:** The truth is that some babies will sleep for a long period of time at night without a feed from the very early weeks and others won't do this until toddlerhood. Those are the extreme ends of the spectrum, and I would say that, on average, most babies can sleep 'through the night' at between six and twelve months. What is classed as 'through the night' also varies wildly depending on who you are talking to. I class it as eight hours plus. Strictly speaking, none of us 'sleep through' without stirring – we cycle between light and deep sleep throughout the night. What we actually mean is that the baby does this without assistance from their parents. This comes with time and practice.

### Q: I'm totally exhausted and not sure where to even start changing my six-month-old's sleep. Help!

**A:** Take a deep breath and make a plan. Start small by aiming to begin your day at roughly the same time each day. This should give you a good idea of the naptimes that work well for your baby. You could aim for a morning nap around two hours after waking (this is a rough guide as some will need it sooner and some a little later) and then another nap two hours after that. Your baby might need a third nap, particularly if the second nap is fairly short. All naps should be finished by 5pm at the latest, if you are aiming for a 7pm bedtime.

### Q: When can I drop all night feeds?

**A:** It's impossible to give a precise age when you should drop all night feeds or hazard a guess as to when your baby no longer requires them. It is so individual. There are also times when your baby might not have had a night feed for several weeks, but you end up needing to give one again. There really is no right or wrong and it varies so much from baby to baby. Many parents find that by around the age of six months their baby has fallen into a rhythm where they will be able to go through without a feed, but it's absolutely not a rule. I have known many babies continue to have one to two night feeds for longer than this, while others drop all night feeds sooner.

### Q: Can I use a dummy just for naps?

**A:** No, if you are using a dummy, you should use it for all sleep times. Offer it at the beginning of each sleep time, day and night. This is due to research around dummy use and SIDS (see page 50). The NHS advice is to remove the dummy at some point between six and twelve months. This is to avoid potential problems that have been identified, such as misalignment of teeth, impact on speech and ear infections. If you do want to get rid of the dummy, then I advise going cold turkey. (For more on dummy use and ditching the dummy, see pages 121 and 161.)

### Q: My ten-month-old baby is waking earlier and earlier. Last week it was 5am and it's now 4.30am! He is happy and full of beans and ready to start the day, but I'm not. Help! What can I do?

**A:** As your little one is waking happy, it is likely that he has simply slept enough. In this instance, you could try a later bedtime. I would do this gradually across the course of a few days – pushing bedtime on by five to ten minutes each day. It is also possible that something in your baby's environment is waking him, so check for any external noises and, if it is summertime, make sure his room is blacked out. You might also assess his morning nap – sometimes if they have a too long or too early morning nap that they no longer need, it can cause early waking.

**Q: My newborn baby is sleeping really well overnight and has returned to his birth weight. Do I need to wake to feed him at night?**

**A:** As long as your baby has returned to his birth weight, and is otherwise healthy and thriving, you don't need to wake him to feed during the night. I would continue to wake him regularly through-out the day (if he naps for longer than two hours), as you don't want him to miss a feed during the day. Keep an eye on the number of wet and dirty nappies he is producing in a 24-hour period.

**Q: I want to work on sleep, but I am worried about crying.**

**A:** Take a step back and work out what you are worried about. If it is leaving your baby alone, you don't have to do this. Choose a grad-ual, gentle method. You might start with 'fade it out' (see page 173). If you think your baby would be better suited to a form of con-trolled crying (see page 182), there are likely to be tears, but, until you try, you don't know how your baby will react or how you will feel. It is always okay to give it a go and then change your mind. You don't have to do anything you don't want to do – perhaps just assess routine and sleep environment first and see how things go.

**Q: We have a great routine and my baby sleeps through the night. What shall I do when the clocks change?**

**A:** You have a few options. You could choose to do nothing and, on the morning of the change, adapt to the new time. You could alternatively move bedtime by 30 minutes the night before either forward or backward depending on if it's the spring (when the clocks go forward) or the autumn (when the clocks go back). The other option is to move bedtime by 15-minute increments in the days leading up to the change. If you do this, be mindful that you need to move your baby's entire day (meals and feeds, for example) too.

### Q: Should I change my baby's nappy in the night if it's not dirty?

**A:** No, modern nappies are very absorbent. If it's just a wee, you should be able to leave it until the morning, unless the nappy is very full. If it is soiled, I would change it with minimal fuss and hopefully settle baby back off to sleep. Keep an eye on your baby's skin as you don't want them to get sore overnight. A good barrier cream can help, but obviously we should always change nappies if they need changing.

### Q: My baby wakes up chatting in the night. Should I leave her?

**A:** If your baby is happy and content in her sleep space, I would leave her to it. Sometimes we rush in when our babies don't need us and stimulate and disturb them. It's a positive thing that your baby is happy in her own company. If this wakeful period is going on for a long time, it could be worth reassessing the amount of daytime sleep she is having. It could be that she is sleeping too much during the day and is therefore very wakeful at night.

### Q: I have tried controlled crying, but my baby just laughs instead of settling. What shall I do?

**A:** It is good to hear that your baby isn't upset by you going in and out of the room. Given this, I would stay out for as long as it takes for your baby to fall asleep. As with any of these methods, they are not set in stone. React to your baby in the moment – if they are happy, you can just stay out of the room. If your baby is very play-ful, maybe they are not ready for bed yet. You could try moving bedtime 10–15 minutes later to see if that has a positive impact.

### Q: Is it bad that my baby feeds to sleep?

**A:** Absolutely not. It is never bad – it's not a rod for your back or any of the other things you may have heard. Feeding to sleep can be a useful tool. You only need to change this if it is not working anymore, for you or for baby.

### Q: How can I stop my baby crawling around the cot?

**A:** It is very common for babies to practise their new-found skills at night-time or naptime in their sleep space and is nothing to worry about. You should allow them the space to do this, and to find their own comfortable sleeping position. If we try to intervene, we can disrupt the process of them settling themselves. Of course, if your baby is upset, you can try the settling methods I have detailed in the book, but crawling around in itself is nothing to worry about.

### Q: Should a pre-nap routine be the same as a bedtime routine?

**A:** I tend to advise doing a 'mini' version of bedtime at naptime. For some babies, being rushed into bed for their nap is jarring. Others will be fine without too much ceremony. You can experi-ment and see what works for your baby, but potentially a nappy change, a change of sleepsuit, then into a sleeping bag and a lul-laby or story works well.

### Q: Is it okay to finish a nap in the pram if my baby wakes up in their cot unhappy?

**A:** Yes, this is absolutely fine. Many families will continue a nap in a different way if their baby wakes up between sleep cycles and is still tired.

## Q: Is ten months too young to drop to one nap per day?

**A:** Every baby is different, but no it is not too young. Most babies will drop to one nap between the ages of ten and eighteen months. If your little one is not settling for their nap anymore or waking very early, these can be good indicators that it is time to reduce or cut the morning nap and have one longer nap in the middle of the day.

## Q: What is the best age to start a routine?

**A:** A gentle rhythm to your day can start in the early weeks, but 'routine' really comes into play later. Any routine you follow should be adapted to and suit your baby. It is not about forcing them into a box. Everyone is different – some people start a gentle routine from six weeks for example, while others might not even consider it until six months.

## Q: Can I feed on demand and work on sleep?

**A:** Absolutely. We can always feed our babies responsively. Sleep work should never be about withholding feeds.

## Q: Can I work on sleep if I haven't moved baby into her own room?

**A:** Yes, absolutely. It might just be that you try a method where you are always with baby or, if your baby is over six months and you have decided to use a controlled crying method (see page 182), that you start this at bedtime when you are not in the room. You can leave the room during the night if you like or revert to an in-the-room settling method.

## Q: What age do babies stop needing a bottle before bed?

**A:** The NHS advises that babies switch to a cup, rather than bottle, of milk before bed at the age of one. I believe we should be practical and not put too much stress on doing this the day they turn one, but to have it in mind to start phasing out bottles. I advise dropping the morning bottle first and going straight to breakfast, then the mid-afternoon one (if your baby has one), replacing that with a snack and drink. I would drop the bedtime bottle last and replace with a cup of milk during story time.

### Q: Is it true that sleep breeds sleep?

**A:** No, this makes no logical sense. I think the belief stems from parents noticing that when their baby is napping 'well' (for example, without parental support), they tend to also sleep well at night – this is down to them settling independently, not down to the amount of sleep they have had. There is only so much sleep any one person can have in a 24-hour period. We can't change someone's sleep requirements. We can only influence 'where' they take that sleep – for example, they might have longer naps and shorter overnight sleep.

### Q: My baby snores a lot – is that normal?

**A:** It is normal for a baby to 'mouth breathe' when they have a cold due to being congested, but if you are ever concerned about your baby's breathing patterns, please consult your doctor. If it is regular snoring, please get this checked out. You can make a video of the snoring to show your doctor or health visitor.

### Q: Do you believe a breastfed baby can use feeds just for comfort, rather than hunger?

**A:** Yes, but there's nothing wrong with that as it is often a very convenient way to settle them. However, if you are feeding very often at night and your baby's satiation feels unsustainable, you can work on new sleep associations. See the advice in Chapter 8.

### Q: Can I work on sleep without any crying?

**A:** I would never make that promise to a parent. Babies cry to communicate with us and we would never want to stop that happening. If we are changing behaviours around bedtime, there is likely to be some upset (although not always!). Depending on your baby's temperament, the method you choose and the speed you do it with, it is possible that there could be minimal crying.

### Q: Why do different sleep consultants have different suggested wake windows?

**A:** I am afraid that 'wake windows' are not an exact science. They are based on what sleep consultants have noticed over the years; this is why I say to take them with a pinch of salt. Working out your baby's individual wake window is best, as they can really vary from baby to baby. For more on wake windows, see page 111.

### Q: My baby settles for naps, but at bedtime he just screams. What should I do?

**A:** It could be that your baby is napping for too long in the day and isn't tired enough at bedtime. I would reassess his naps and timings. Perhaps also consider his bedtime routine – is there enough time for some connection with you before bed? Or are you rushing bedtime?

### Q: Should I cap my baby's morning nap?

**A:** It really depends on your baby. Sometimes we need to do this to protect the next nap or to protect against early waking. However, some babies are happier having a longer morning nap. If it works well for your family, you don't need to cap it.

### Q: Do babies need their hands covered at night?

**A:** In most cases, no. I only tend to cover them if they have bad eczema (see page 263). Otherwise, I think it is good to allow babies access to their hands in order to settle themselves.

## Q: My baby was sleeping well, but now she's not. Is it a regression?

**A:** Read Chapter 7 on the 'four-to-six-month sleep progression'. This will tell you all you need to know.

## Q: How many naps does my baby need?

**A:** This very much depends on your baby's age and how long their naps are. At around three to six months, most babies take three naps. The third nap tends to be dropped by around eight months (or earlier) and the second nap is dropped between ten and eighteen months. The last nap can remain up to the age of four, although many will drop it between the ages of two and three years old. If your baby is having very short naps, then of course they could be more frequent. And if they are having very long naps, then they will be less frequent. This is just a rough guide. We also need to consider their amount of daytime sleep – if they are waking up at 6am they are going to have a different sleep requirement to a baby who wakes at 7.30am, for example.

## Q: My baby won't take a long lunchtime nap. What can I do?

**A:** Don't panic. Nothing bad will happen if they don't have a long nap at lunchtime. Your baby can have another nap later or you can work on your timings. It might be that you need to push this nap a little later so that their sleep pressure builds a bit more. Alternatively, it could be that working on how they settle at naptime naturally extends this nap.

## Q: I have tried controlled crying, but I feel that the crying is too much for me and for my baby. What else can I do?

**A:** Take a step back and reassess. Don't worry if it is not for you. Have a look at Chapter 8 and pick a slower method.

**Q: I have chosen the method where I fade out sleep associations, but our progress is so slow it has barely changed anything. What can I do?**

**A:** You could be in this for the long haul – this method can be really effective, but you need to make sure you are keeping up with gradual changes. If we don't change anything, we can't expect to see change.

**Q: How can I fit feeding solids into my six-month-old's routine?**

**A:** This is when routine really becomes important and I believe it is helpful to work towards predictable mealtimes. When your baby first starts solids, they will only be on one meal, and will build up to three meals gradually over the coming months. Most people start with a breakfast or a lunch, but there's no rule to it – do whatever works best for you and your baby.

**Q: My baby is poorly with a virus, so should I stop working on changing her sleep? And how long should I let her nap?**

**A:** I would pause your plan and return to it when your baby is better. Go with the flow when it comes to naps. If your baby has slept a lot more than usual during the day and is very wakeful at night for long periods of time, maybe consider capping naps the next day, or when she is well again.

**Q: Do I need to give up breastfeeding to work on sleep?**

**A:** Absolutely not. Your feeding method has very little to do with sleep long term. Breast milk and first infant formula are almost identical in terms of calories, but also research tells us that the waking patterns of babies are similar in both breastfed and formula-fed babies. Working on your baby's sleep does not need to involve switching feeding method unless you want to. Breast milk does include some hormones that can help your baby fall asleep, and breastfeeding is certainly not a barrier to a good night's sleep.

### Q: I have a toddler and a baby. How do I manage bedtime with both?

**A:** It can be challenging when you have more than one child to attend to, especially if you are doing the bedtime routine on your own. Organisation is key. Bathing your baby and toddler together is helpful – try to have everything you need ready in the bathroom. Give the baby a very short dip in the bath and get them dressed in the bathroom while your toddler is splashing around. Then get your toddler out and dressed while your baby lies on a playmat in the bathroom. Then all head to the toddler's bedroom together and feed your baby there while your toddler chooses a book. If you are able to, you could read to your toddler while you feed or have a quiet activity set up for your toddler. Then settle your baby down and return to your toddler for some special one-to-one time and an extra story.

### Q: What should I say to family members who criticise my baby's routine?

**A:** It can be tricky when you are faced with criticism. The best thing is to stay calm and measured in your response. Try to explain why what you are doing benefits you and your baby. If they still don't understand, try using some of the methods on page 44.

### Q: I really want to change my baby's sleep habits, but I am worried that it won't work and I will fail.

**A:** The fear of failure can be a real roadblock to many parents. Don't think of the things I speak about in this book as 'working' or 'not working'. Consider the information to be things that you can try out, experiment with, and see how you get on. You will not fail, as there is no exam to pass – it's just about helping your baby to sleep a bit better.

# USEFUL RESOURCES

**Association of Breastfeeding Mothers (ABM)**
https://abm.me.uk/
Helpline: 0300 330 5453

**Association of Tongue-Tie Practitioners (ATP)**
Find a practitioner.
https://www.tongue-tie.org.uk/find-a-practitioner/

**Baby Sling Safety**
The UK Sling Consortium T.I.C.K.S rules for safe baby-wearing.
https://babyslingsafety.co.uk/

**Cry-sis**
Support for crying and sleepless babies.
https://www.cry-sis.org.uk/
Helpline: 08451 228 669

**Lactation Consultants of Great Britain (LCGB)**
Find an IBCLC lactation consultant near you.
https://lcgb.org/find-an-ibclc/

**La Leche League**
Breastfeeding support from pregnancy onwards.
https://www.laleche.org.uk/
Helpline: 0345 120 2918

## The Lullaby Trust

A charity that raises awareness of sudden infant death syndrome
(SIDS), provides expert advice on safer sleep for babies and
offers emotional support for bereaved families.
https://www.lullabytrust.org.uk/

## Mind

Mental health charity.
https://www.mind.org.uk/
Infoline: 0300 123 3393

## National Breastfeeding Helpline

Breastfeeding information and support.
https://www.nationalbreastfeedinghelpline.org.uk/
Helpline: 0300 100 0212

## National Childbirth Trust (NCT)

https://www.nct.org.uk/
Helpline: 0300 330 0700

## National Deaf Children's Society

Supporting deaf children.
https://www.ndcs.org.uk/

## NHS

Information on vitamins for children.
https://www.nhs.uk/conditions/baby/weaning-and-feeding/
vitamins-for-children/

## PANDAS

Postnatal depression awareness and support.
https://pandasfoundation.org.uk/
Helpline: 0808 1961 776

**Pelvic Partnership**

Information about pelvic girdle pain (PGP).

https://pelvicpartnership.org.uk/

**Refuge**

For women and children. Against domestic violence.

https://refuge.org.uk/

Helpline: 0808 2000 247

**Samaritans**

https://www.samaritans.org/

Helpline: 116 123

**Steps Charity**

For anyone affected by a lower limb problem.

https://www.stepsworldwide.org/

**Twins Trust**

For information on support and networking.

https://twinstrust.org/

**Women's Aid**

Working to provide life-saving services and build a future where domestic violence is not tolerated.

https://www.womensaid.org.uk/

**Facebook support groups for hip spica**

There are a number of Facebook pages about hip spica – have a look at these ones to start:

- DDH – Hip Dysplasia – Children Facing Surgery or Spica Casts (closed group and forum)
- DDH UK Because Hips Matter

- DDH UK Forum and Support Group
- DDH Hip Dysplasia – Children facing surgery or spica casts

**The Royal Society for Blind Children**

Supporting a life without limits for blind children.

https://www.rsbc.org.uk/

**Microphthalmia, Anophthalmia & Coloboma Support**

Supporting children born without eyes or with underdeveloped eyes.

https://macs.org.uk/

# NOTES

## CHAPTER 2: THE TRANSFORMATIVE POWER OF SLEEP

1 Spruyt, K., Aitken, R.J., So, K., Charlton, M., Adamson, T.M. and Horne, R.S., 'Relationship between sleep/wake patterns, temperament and overall development in term infants over the first year of life.' *Early Human Development* 84(5) (2008): 289–96.

## CHAPTER 4: GETTING THE BASICS RIGHT

1 Papalambros, N.A., Santostasi, G., Malkani, R.G., Braun, R., Weintraub, S., Paller, K.A. and Zee, P.C., 'Acoustic enhancement of sleep slow oscillations and concomitant memory improvement in older adults.' *Frontiers in Human Neuroscience* (2017): 109.

2 UK Sling Consortium, 'The T.I.C.K.S. rule for safe babywearing.' Baby Sling Safety (2015). Retrieved from http://babyslingsafety.co.uk.

## CHAPTER 5: THE FOURTH TRIMESTER

1 Iranpour, S., Kheirabadi, G.R., Esmaillzadeh, A., Heidari-Beni, M. and Maracy, M.R., 'Association between sleep quality and postpartum depression.' *Journal of Research in Medical Sciences* 21 (2016): 110.

## CHAPTER 6: FINDING YOUR RHYTHM

1 Yates, J., 'PERSPECTIVE: The long-term effects of light exposure on establishment of newborn circadian rhythm.' *Journal of Clinical Sleep Medicine* 14(10) (2018): 1829–30.

2 Hanafin, S. and Griffiths, P. 'Does pacifier use cause ear infections in young children?' Heal Research Board, Ireland. DOI: 10.12968/ bjcn.2002.7.4.10227.

## CHAPTER 7: THE FOUR-TO-SIX-MONTH 'PROGRESSION'

1   Brown, A. and Harries, V., 'Infant sleep and night feeding patterns during later infancy: Association with breastfeeding frequency, daytime complementary food intake, and infant weight.' *Breastfeeding Medicine* 10(5) (2015): 246–52.

2   Boyce, W.T., *The Orchid and the Dandelion: Why sensitive people struggle and how all can thrive* (Bluebird, 2020).

3   Shaughnessy, A.F., 'Getting an infant to sleep: Graduated extinction and sleep fading are effective.' *American Family Physician* 94(9) (2016): 750.

4   Woodhouse, S.S., Scott, J.R., Hepworth, A.D. and Cassidy, J., 'Secure base provision: A new approach to examining links between maternal caregiving and infant attachment.' *Child Development* 91(1) (2020): e249–65.

5   Hiscock, H., Bayer, J., Gold, L., Hampton, A., Ukoumunne, O.C. and Wake, M., 'Improving infant sleep and maternal mental health: A cluster randomised trial.' *Archives of Disease in Childhood* 92(11) (2007): 952–8.

6   Eckerberg, B., 'Treatment of sleep problems in families with young children: Effects of treatment on family well-being.' *Acta Paediatrica* 93(1) (2004): 126–34.

7   Park, J., Kim, S.Y. and Lee, K., 'Effectiveness of behavioral sleep interventions on children's and mothers' sleep quality and maternal depression: A systematic review and meta-analysis.' *Scientific Reports* 12(1) (2022): 1–11.

8   https://scholarworks.smith.edu/theses/588/.

## CHAPTER 11: SLEEP AND RELATIONSHIPS

1   Kahn, M., Barnett, N. and Gradisar, M., 'Let's talk about sleep baby: Sexual activity postpartum and its links with room sharing, parent sleep, and objectively measured infant sleep and parent nighttime crib visits.' *The Journal of Sex Research* (2022): 1–12.

# ACKNOWLEDGEMENTS

To my beautiful children, without you this book would never have happened, and I wouldn't do what I do. I would never have known what true tiredness is, learned to find my way out of it, and taught others how to do the same.

My husband, Dan – when the world feels dark you are always my shining light. Thank you for supporting me to get these words onto paper. I truly couldn't have done any of it without your love and understanding.

Thank you, Dad – for always telling me the truth, without sugar-coating it. The voice of reason when I am being unreasonable. My mum – for loving me always, and never failing to tell me that everything changes, and nothing stays the same.

I wasn't sure I would ever write a book, but the right people came into my life at the right time. Thank you to my agent Becca for being at the end of the phone and for your invaluable guidance. Thank you to Sam Jackson and the team at Penguin – you helped me to bring these words to life.

And ultimately, thank you to anyone who has ever followed me on social media, shared one of my posts or told a tired friend about me. Not only have you helped more people get the sleep they deserve, but you have helped give me a platform to keep spreading the word. Even on the longest of nights, there is always hope and good sleep on the horizon.

Love Rosey x

# INDEX

Note: page numbers in **bold** refer to diagrams, page numbers in *italics* refer to information contained in tables.